ALLEN CARR'S
EASY WAY
FOR WOMEN TO
QUIT
SMOKING

ALLEN CARR'S
EASY WAY
FOR WOMEN TO
QUIT
SMOKING

SIRIUS

ALLEN CARR

In 1983, after countless failed attempts to cure his own addiction to nicotine, Allen Carr discovered what the world had been waiting for – the easy way to stop smoking. After giving up a successful career as an accountant to help cure the world's smokers, he built a global reputation as a result of his phenomenal method as well as a network of clinics spanning the world. *Allen Carr's Easy Way to Stop Smoking* became an international bestseller and has been published in more than 40 different languages.

In 1998 Allen Carr was invited to speak at the 10th World Conference on Tobacco and Health, held in Beijing, an honour that the most eminent physician would be proud of. His method and reputation could receive no higher commendation. He was widely accepted as the world's leading expert on how to help smokers quit.

The success of Easyway encouraged people with other problems to approach Allen for help. After tests with some of his patients, it was discovered that the simple logic of Easyway also worked well for people with a drink problem, and so Allen wrote *Easy Way to Control Alcohol.* The Easyway method has since been applied to areas such as over-eating, gambling, over-spending, worrying and fear of flying.

A full list of Allen Carr centres appears at the back of this book. Should you require any assistance, do not hesitate to contact your nearest therapist. For futher information, go to **www.allencarr.com**.

Men are from Mars

My special thanks to the female therapists
at my centres, for smoothing the rough edges and for
incorporating the Venus touch.

SIRIUS

This edition published in 2018 by Sirius Publishing, a division of
Arcturus Publishing Limited,
26/27 Bickels Yard, 151–153 Bermondsey Street,
London SE1 3HA

ISBN: 978-1-78888-129-6
AD000031UK

Printed in the USA

CONTENTS

INTRODUCTION

'You'll end up like him!'

I still hear my mother's voice from years ago. I see her pointing in the direction of a frail, seated man, older than his years, panting and coughing in the corner. That man was my father, reduced to a shadow of his former self by emphysema and chronic bronchitis. I would look at him without really seeing him: a few minutes later, I would open the window of my room, inhaling, along with the wintry dampness, the first puffs of yet another cigarette.

I had started smoking twenty years earlier: twenty years of lies, fears, and various attempts to stop – all of which failed. Twenty years timed by the pendulum that swings in every smoker's mind:

'Oh, my God! What is this twinge in my throat – I've got to quit… soon.' *Tick.*

'Now isn't the right time to quit.' *Tock.*

'Damn! I forgot the cigarettes! I've got to go out again.' *Tick.*

'I'll quit when this stressful period is over!' *Tock.*

And the pendulum would have carried on, *tick-tock-tick-tock,* until the inevitable and unthinkable end. But a year later, in London – where I was living at the time – a lady gave me a telephone number, saying, 'My husband, who was a chain-smoker, went to see this gentleman named Allen Carr. Since then, my husband hasn't touched a cigarette, and he is as happy as a clam!'

A few days later, I found myself among a group of fellow smokers in the presence of this Mr Carr. Everywhere were copies of his book and mountains of letters, all with the same message: 'Thank you, Allen Carr! Your book/your seminar has saved me/ freed me/changed my life forever…'

Initially sceptical and petrified, I listened to Allen talk. Every sentence slowly unscrewed the pendulum's devices, revealing its sinister mechanism. Word after word, I began to understand the mental associations and the traps that had been the bars of my prison for more than twenty-one years. Now, contrary to my view of my father, I was not only looking, but I was able to see – and everything was so clear, so ridiculously obvious and easy!

A few short hours later, I realized that the pendulum was actually silent. It had finally stopped!

Allen Carr held his first seminar in 1983; by 1985, purely on the strength of word-of-mouth recommendations, he had become unable to cope with the number of smokers seeking his help. His solution was to put his method into a book. The book has now sold more than 12 million copies worldwide. Allen Carr's lasting legacy is not only a dynamic ongoing publishing programme, but also a network of stop-smoking clinics that spans the globe.

Ten years after I sat in that room with Allen Carr, it was my huge privilege to introduce Allen Carr's Easyway to Stop Smoking Seminars to my father's homeland, Italy. It was my honour and joy to work so closely with the man who had freed me from my addiction to nicotine. In 2003, I was entrusted to translate and publish the book in Italy, where, as in so many other countries, it remained a top-ten bestseller for many years. Getting involved in this way was the least I could do: helping others to free themselves was enormously gratifying. There are now over 150 Allen Carr's Easyway centres in more than forty-five countries. Each centre was established by people like me who had found it easy and exhilarating to quit smoking after reading the book or participating in a seminar. We have each decided to join the organization to bring Allen Carr's Easyway to our own countries.

The book is now a global bestseller, and more than 400,000 smokers have attended Allen Carr's Easyway seminars. The same heartfelt, grateful and moving letters that I saw in London many years ago now arrive on our desks daily from New York, Los Angeles, Toronto, Milan, Tokyo, Madrid, Moscow, Santiago, Berlin, Paris, Sydney, Mexico City, Belgrade, Amsterdam, Dublin, and so on.

I stopped smoking in August 1988, and in the following years I never stopped thanking Allen. Without him, not only would I not be here writing these words, but, most probably, I would not be here at all. THANK YOU, ALLEN!

To have been asked to help Allen address the smoking problem from a female point of view was the biggest compliment that anyone could have paid me.

The number of women smokers is rising inexorably as the number of male smokers is slowly declining. Although Allen Carr's original book works just as well for women as it does for men, women perceive many of the issues associated with smoking differently. After all, men are from Mars and we are from Venus. There are particular difficulties faced by women who want to quit, including those arising from the perceived links between cigarettes and fashion, style, sex, glamour, stress relief, and weight control. Every aspect of smoking is examined from a female perspective, providing answers to female-specific questions and concerns.

I have written about privilege and honour already. Perhaps sometimes we use those words too cheaply, but in this instance I think they are understatements. Helping Allen to apply the Venus touch in channelling his method in this special way has been one of the most exciting, enjoyable, and liberating processes of my life. I am certain that you will find reading this book and the result that it achieves equally spectacular.

It is natural for you to be nervous and sceptical – I remember having those feelings myself all those years ago in London – but read on with an open mind. Allen and I have nothing but good news for you!

Francesca Cesati

FOREWORD

By John Dicey, Global CEO & Senior Therapist,
Allen Carr's Easyway

Allen Carr's Easyway organization is now widely accepted as the world's leading authority on stopping smoking and the method has been successfully applied to alcohol, weight issues, fear of flying, gambling, debt, sugar addiction, caffeine addiction, and a whole host of legal and illegal drugs.

I'm aware that the claims of the method's success might appear far-fetched or exaggerated, at times even outrageous. That was certainly my reaction when I first heard them. I was incredibly fortunate to attend Allen Carr's clinic in London in 1997, yet I did so under duress. I had agreed to go, at the request of my wife, on the understanding that when I walked out of the clinic and remained a smoker she would leave it at least 12 months before hassling me about stopping smoking again. No one was more surprised than me, or perhaps my wife, that Allen Carr's Easyway method set me free from my 80-a-day addiction.

I was so inspired that I hassled and harangued Allen Carr and Robin Hayley (now Chairman of Allen Carr's Easyway) to let me get involved in their quest to cure the world of smoking. I was incredibly fortunate to have succeeded in convincing them to allow me to do so. Being trained by Allen Carr and Robin Hayley was one of the most rewarding experiences of my life. To be able to count Allen as not only my coach and mentor but also my friend was an amazing honour and privilege. Allen Carr and Robin Hayley trained me well – I went on to personally treat more than 30,000 smokers at Allen's original London centre, and became part of the team that has taken Allen's method from Berlin to Bogota, from New Zealand to New York, from Sydney to Santiago. Tasked by Allen with ensuring that his legacy achieves its full potential, we've taken Allen Carr's Easyway from videos to DVD, from clinics to apps, from computer games to audio books, to online programs, video-on-demand and beyond.

The honour of adding a light editorial touch in the form of a foreword to this book has fallen to me. This enables us to look at issues such as e-cigarettes that have emerged in recent years and, in fact, to look at the use of all forms of nicotine. Please bear with me as you read this short but important foreword – believe me, it's important to do so whether you're a user of e-cigarettes or other nicotine products, or not. I promise to leave you in Allen Carr's safe hands after that.

Whether you're a cigarette, cigar, or pipe smoker, or a vaper (user of e-cigarettes), nicotine patch wearer, nicotine gum chewer, nicotine inhalator, snus, or dip user – in fact a user of nicotine via any delivery device available – this book will set you free.

If you've never vaped or used other nicotine devices, you might make the mistake of thinking this section of the book simply doesn't apply to you. Don't! The rest of this book will enable you to find it ridiculously easy to stop smoking – you'll never have to suffer with nicotine addiction again. But to avoid falling back into the nicotine trap in the future, you must understand it completely.

You're escaping from the torture of nicotine addiction, not just escaping from smoking. If you don't understand nicotine addiction, there is always a danger that perhaps in the future you might try an e-cigarette just to see what it's like. If you do, you'll fall right back into the trap. This is particularly important as e-cigarettes, or whatever the next new-fangled nicotine product might be, are subject to ruthless marketing

One of the most powerful and influential marketing machines on the planet is ramping up its activities once again. Their target? You and your kids! This book will set you free, just as other Easyway titles have done for tens of millions before you, but one puff of a cigarette, cigar, pipe, 'joint' with tobacco, e-cigarette, or intake of nicotine by any means will trap you again. Understand why you need to avoid all nicotine and you will not only be set free forever, but find it ridiculously easy to stop and, more importantly, stay stopped.

You'd have thought that the people who claimed that nicotine addiction, in the form of cigarette smoking, could be cured by giving the addict nicotine in the form of patches and gum would retreat in shame once the folly of their claim was exposed by its spectacular failure to so. This, in spite of huge amounts of taxpayers' money being spent on the scheme.

However, they concluded that the problem with their plan was that the addicts didn't receive a big enough dose of nicotine, frequently enough, or quickly enough, when they used patches or gum. They also decided that rather than nicotine being capable of curing nicotine addiction the best they could hope for was for the addict to remain addicted to nicotine in the long term – hopefully ingesting the substance in a less harmful way.

As time passes, and the inconvenient truth emerges that, far from helping smokers to quit, e-cigarettes actually help them to carry on smoking, these people continue to ignore Allen Carr's Easyway: a safe, inexpensive, proven cure for smoking that requires no drugs of any sort, let alone nicotine.

There is no doubt that some people have quit smoking while using e-cigarettes, yet they have done so in spite of them, rather than because of them.

Even for those few who might become solely addicted to e-cigarettes instead of smoking, there remains a number of significantly negative factors for addicts and their families if they stay addicted to nicotine.

The last thing most smokers are worried about is the money; yet it's worth just pausing for a moment to assess who the winners and losers are with regard to the nicotine industry.

In 2014, the cost to the UK National Health Service caused by smoking was £2 billion a year ($2.5bn) , with the cost of social care for older smokers being around £1.1 billion ($1.5bn) a year. That's a combined cost of £3.1 billion ($4bn) a year.

UK tax revenue from tobacco excise and VAT around that time

was £12.3 billion ($16.3bn) a year! That's a benefit to Her Majesty's Treasury of more than £9 billion ($12bn) a year!

Yet smokers are bullied, and harassed, and made to feel like outcasts by a system that views them as a ready-made profit centre. As nicotine addiction in other forms grows, you can be sure that the Treasury will be ready to apply the same taxes to those products. What more predictable and sustainable source of income is there than an addict?

As a nicotine addict you have to ask yourself: do you really want to be a victim of this scam any longer? Can it really be that the governments of the world are disincentivized from curing nicotine addiction and might even be happy to encourage it?

Global corporations such as Microsoft, Vodafone, IBM, Ford, Total, Esso, Pfizer, and BMW, to name but a few, contract our services for to help their employees stop smoking.

They do it, not just because they're fabulous employers who care about their people, but also because it saves them around £4,000 ($5,270) a year for each employee who quits smoking (lost productivity, increased sickness, etc.). The more smokers we cure, the more money they save (and we provide our money-back guarantee, so they really can't lose).

Every time a smoker quits, it costs the government money in lost tax revenue for the duration of the former smoker's life. If you've wondered why the government don't use our services, then within the last few paragraphs there's a clue or two as to why not.

Can you see how governments might be financially disincentivized to help smokers, vapers, or any kind of nicotine addict escape?

The e-cigarette manufacturers are not just interested in convincing smokers to switch to vaping; they also shamelessly target youngsters. Who do you think they're trying to appeal to with flavours such as bubble-gum, gummy bears, fruit loops, skittles, cotton candy, and popcorn?

Of course the nicotine industry is rubbing its hands with glee. Get the addicts younger and you maximize the lifetime income per user. One can only assume that Treasury departments feel likewise.

A certain number of kids have always tried out cigarettes, but the way e-cigarettes are creeping into everyday life is something else. It's creating a new gateway into smoking and nicotine addiction.

You can imagine how the kids get sucked in. Firstly, the peer pressure to move on to 'the real thing' is already there, but more significantly there's the fact that no e-cigarette will ever deliver nicotine as efficiently as a cigarette. All addicts eventually end up looking for ways to get more of their drug into their bloodstream faster, and so it is with nicotine. That's where cigarettes come in.

Studies are continually confirming that the vast majority of e-cigarette users continue to smoke rather than quit completely. They never achieve the reduced harm they dreamed of when they started using e-cigarettes and end up taking in more nicotine, rather than less, as a result. At times when they would previously have abstained from smoking altogether, they now vape.

Now, if you're one of the few e-cigarette or other nicotine product users who have successfully stopped smoking but remain hooked on nicotine, you're very much the exception. For you the advantages of becoming entirely free from nicotine remain compelling; after all, isn't that why you're reading this book? So please, don't be offended by our assertion that the vast majority of e-cigarette users continue to smoke; it happens to be true. While you continue to be addicted to nicotine, you remain vulnerable to smoking and all the downsides of addiction. Getting free from those is priceless.

In summary then, we have a new generation of addicts in development. Existing smokers are likely to be increasing their intake of nicotine rather than decreasing it (by smoking AND vaping); there continues to be a re-normalization of smoker/ smoker-like behaviour; many former smokers are being drawn back into nicotine addiction and smoking. Little is known of the health effects of long-term nicotine use in the dual form of smoking and vaping (or just vaping, for that matter); and those with a vested interest in 'The Nicotine Industry' will lead the field in establishing how harmful or otherwise it may turn out to be. And we all know how well that's turned out in the past!

This is an industry with a proven track record of fraud on a global scale, built on lies, bribery, corruption, suppression of study data that's resulted in tens of millions of lives being lost, direct involvement in organized international tobacco smuggling, aggressive marketing to children in the developing world, as well as more covert targeting of youngsters in other parts of the world where direct marketing to children is forbidden. This is the most powerful and destructive industry on the planet. And they appear to be winning 'The Nicotine War'.

You don't want to be a casualty or victim of that war; that's why you're reading this book. As Allen Carr guides you through his amazing method over the coming chapters, he talks exclusively about cigarettes. In doing so, he's really referring to nicotine in all its forms.

Carry on smoking, vaping, or smoking AND vaping, as you read the book; don't be tempted to cut down or control your intake as you read.

But if you haven't smoked a cigarette for a long period, there's no need for you to do so. At the end of the book, when you're asked to have a final cigarette or e-cigarette, just confirm in your mind that you've already done so.

In the unlikely event that you've vaped without smoking for a long period, just carry on vaping as you read. You'll still be able to relate virtually all of the text to your vaping. Please do make sure that you do that as you read. The same goes for you if you are using patches, gum, snus, dip, or nicotine in any form.

When it comes to the final cigarette at the end of the book, just have one final e-cigarette or shot of nicotine in whatever form you've been using it.

Follow Allen Carr's instructions and you'll find it not only easy to be free, but you'll actually enjoy the whole process of quitting. You won't just be free, you'll be happy to be free. That might sound too good to be true at the moment, but read on. You've got nothing to lose and absolutely everything to gain. Let me pass you into the safest of hands – over to Allen Carr.

1 *Ladies First*

After generations of servitude Western women are finally achieving equality, not only in the work-place, where they are now represented at the highest levels even in previously male-dominated professions, but in all other areas of life. Few people would dispute this and many would say, 'about time too'. By far the most important aspect of this success to me in relation to answering the question of why women smoke is how the great pioneers of the movement for equality won the argument.

These women dared to challenge the prevailing perceptions and rules. They refused to accept the situation as being the only possible scenario for society, and put forward compelling reasons for rejecting the stereotypical female roles allotted to them. There were, of course, many women who, while secretly supporting their 'sisters', were too scared to follow this example. Then there were still more who accepted the situation without question.

It is a strange thing but often life's wrongs only become obvious once we do question them. If we don't question, we are accepting the situation, whatever that may be. The brainwashing applies to practically every aspect of our lives. In this book we are initially concerned with just two aspects of the brainwashing: as it relates to smoking itself, and as it relates to the differences between men and women.

My dictionary defines brainwashing as:

'To effect a radical change in the ideas and beliefs of a person.'

You might well ask yourself what all this has to do with stopping smoking. We all know that smoking is a filthy, disgusting habit that ruins our health and wealth. Nowadays even smokers themselves regard it as a decidedly anti-social pastime. So why do you need to alter your views and beliefs in order to stop? Surely there's a magic pill or trick to stop you wanting a cigarette? You might also be wondering how just reading a book could possibly help you to stop. Let me explain how:

What is it that you are actually trying to achieve? That's obvious: to put out your final cigarette and never want to smoke another.

No doubt you know of many ex-smokers who have successfully managed to stop, but didn't most of them have several failed attempts before they succeeded? Even when they did succeed, didn't they have to use considerable willpower together with pills, patches or gum? And didn't they have to suffer days, weeks or months or years of misery? And how many of them still wanted – almost begged you for – an occasional cigarette? I bet you can remember others who have told you that although they prefer being non-smokers, meals and social occasions are not quite as enjoyable without a cigarette, and whenever the telephone rings they find themselves reaching for the packet that no longer exists.

Is this really what you are trying to achieve?

But for the moment just forget about trying never to smoke again. Try to answer this important question: What is the difference between a smoker and a non-smoker?

The answer appears to be obvious: one smokes, the other doesn't. True, but it's not quite as simple as that, is it? No one ever forces you to light up. So do smokers only ever light a cigarette because they want to? Well, no, because you know there are times when you light up not because you want to but purely out of habit. In fact, most twenty-a-day smokers freely admit that they only actually enjoy about two of these cigarettes; the rest are purely habitual. But if this were true, it should be a simple matter to limit ourselves. We could keep our cigarettes in a locked drawer, and this practical impediment to lighting up would enable us to pause for thought when the urge came upon us. As we were thinking about reaching for the key, we could ask ourselves: Am I lighting up to enjoy this smoke, or is it just habitual? If it were simply habitual, there would be little point in smoking that cigarette.

This simple ruse would enable twenty-a-day smokers to reduce to two-a-day without any aggravation whatsoever. If you have tried this or a similar ruse, you will know that it works only for a limited period – that is, until your willpower runs out. Have you ever tried to enlist the help of your children, grandchildren or best friend by putting them in charge of your cigarettes? You will know only too well to what lengths you will go to get those cigarettes back, despite your declarations that your pleas should be ignored when the urge to light up arises. No matter how strong their resolution not to give them back to you, nothing can resist the panic, ingenuity and determination of a smoker who has reached the stage of wanting a cigarette NOW!

Women are renowned for their protective maternal instincts and likewise their sense of retribution if a wrong is done to them. Yet we read horror stories of mothers who leave their children at home to fend for themselves while they have a good time on the town or even abroad. We scorn and ridicule such women for their lack of responsibility. But if you are brutally honest with yourself, can't you recall incidents when you've sneaked out of the house – just for a moment – while the kids were asleep in order to head down to the gas station to buy some cigarettes? Aren't there times when you've left them in the car with the engine running while you popped into the corner store? I even heard of one woman in a maternity ward who was so desperate for a cigarette that she implored an orderly to keep an eye on her newly born baby while she went to get a pack. The over-tasked orderly refused. Needless to say, she was a non-smoker: someone who has never smoked as opposed to an ex-smoker. Her comments – 'You know you don't really need one', 'It's not good for your health or your baby's', and 'You went through a fourteen-hour labour without one' – simply served to compound the woman's guilt. But they didn't stop her going, despite this being just after extensive media coverage of an abduction of a new-born from a hospital. When the mother returned, the baby had gone and the ensuing panic and her screams could be heard throughout the hospital. Fortunately, the baby was in safe hands and had simply been moved to a different ward by another orderly, but imagine how that mother felt in the minutes it took to ascertain the true situation.

I have used this example to illustrate both the effect and power of brainwashing. Just as girls will often criticize their friends for failing to stop when they become pregnant, yet fail to stop themselves when they in turn become pregnant, so it is difficult to believe that the incident I have described could ever happen to a conscientious mother. Before you condemn her, be honest with yourself. Have you never driven miles in search of an all-night garage or store because you'd run out of cigarettes? Have you never experienced the panic feeling that goes with being down to your last few cigarettes or, worst scenario of all, being completely out of cigarettes? Of course you have.

If you could take or leave cigarettes, as many smokers claim, why on earth would you be reading this book? You are reading it for one reason and one reason alone:

FEAR

Don't worry, that's the only reason any smoker continues to smoke. That woman didn't risk her baby because of the pleasure of breathing cancerous fumes into her lungs. She did it because she was in a panic without cigarettes.

Picture a heroin addict with no heroin. Visualize the panic, the shakes, the pain, the fear. Now imagine the relief when the addict is allowed to self-inject heroin into a vein in an arm resembling a dartboard. Do you really believe that heroin addicts enjoy injecting themselves? Non-heroin addicts find it impossible to believe that they can.

Non-smokers find it difficult to believe that smokers actually enjoy breathing lethal fumes into their lungs. So did you before you became hooked on nicotine. I was brainwashed to believe that heroin addicts injected themselves in order to obtain unbelievably pleasurable hallucinations or dreams.

In fact they do it to end the anxious, shaking, insecure feeling they suffer as the drug leaves their body.

One of the many common misconceptions about all drug addiction is that addicts only suffer withdrawal symptoms when they attempt to stop using the drug. In truth they suffer them from the moment the first dose begins to leave their bodies, and the only reason they take the next dose is to try to end the empty, insecure feeling that the previous dose creates.

People who aren't addicted to heroin don't suffer that panic feeling. It's exactly the same with smoking. Non-smokers cannot understand why anyone would even want to breathe those filthy fumes into their lungs, let alone spend a fortune and risk awful diseases in order to do so. And as for risking the life of your baby rather than wait an hour longer – that is not only outrageous but completely incomprehensible to non-smokers. As a fellow addict I couldn't condone that lady's conduct, but I could sympathize with how she had got into that state. It's not particularly pleasant to hold a plastic bag over your head, even when you know you can remove it whenever you want. But it's anathema for someone else to hold it over your head, even someone who loves you, especially if they think they are doing you a favour by doing so.

Let's spend a few moments considering the effects of what I have been saying. I asked you to consider the difference between a smoker and a non-smoker. The obvious answer is that one smokes and the other doesn't. This also happens to be the correct answer, and because it is both obvious and correct, we inadvertently approach the solution to the problem back to front. In other words, we try to solve the problem by never smoking again. This might still seem logical to you at this stage. Let me explain why it is not, by putting a different problem to you.

You have a tile missing from your roof. Every time it rains you are left with a damp patch on your expensive carpet. How do you solve your problem? There are several steps you might take. You could take up your carpet or keep a bucket permanently over the spot to catch the rain, or you might even take the drastic step of moving home. None of these steps would solve your problem, though. The most sensible and cost-effective solution would be to remove the cause of the problem by replacing the missing tile.

There is a tendency to apply the same principle to other problems in our lives. That is, often we choose not to face the underlying causes. If a tyre on your car or bike looks flat, you'd probably hope to solve the problem by having it pumped up. If it's flat again after a few days and you are lazy or an optimist or, like me, you are both, you might have it pumped up again and repeat this process several more times. But no matter how lazy or optimistic we might be, if it goes down a second time we know that we have a slow puncture and that the only solution is to have the tyre fixed.

The real difference between a smoker and a non-smoker is not that one smokes and the other doesn't. The lighting of a cigarette is only the effect of the real problem. To hope to stop smoking by never smoking another cigarette is equivalent to permanently keeping a bucket under the hole in your roof rather than replacing the tile, or having to pump up your bicycle tyre every few days rather than fix the puncture.

The real difference between a smoker and a non-smoker is that a smoker has a need or desire to smoke and a non-smoker does not. That is the real problem: the equivalent to the missing tile or the slow puncture. Just accept this indisputable fact: nobody but ourselves forces us to light up. Even when others move heaven and earth to prevent us from doing so, we'll find a way of preventing them. Also accept the indisputable fact that, even when we are trying to cut down or to stop permanently, the only difficulty is that another part of our brain is saying 'But I want a cigarette!' If this were not true, 'giving up' smoking would be easy. You might find this difficult to believe, but stopping smoking is easy for any smoker, including you, providing you go about it the right way.

So, in order to stop smoking we need to solve the problem at source: we need to remove the need or desire to smoke, not just for a few hours, days, months or years, but permanently. Even the authorities find it difficult to believe that it is possible to stop smoking without the use of an ounce of willpower. But just think about it – if you never had the need or desire to light up another cigarette, why would you need willpower not to do so?

You might well be thinking: 'This is all very well and I cannot dispute what you say. In fact, I cannot but accept that, because no one but me forces me to smoke, there must be some self-destructive flaw in my make-up. But how can a book possibly remove that flaw?'

EUREKA! You've hit the nub of the problem. With the missing tile and the slow puncture, we can see clearly both the cause of the problem and the solution. With smoking we can see clearly that the solution is to remove the desire to smoke – permanently. Easily said, but how do we do that?

We have to go a stage further. Before we can remove this need or desire to smoke, we need to understand why we have it. After all, we weren't born with it. The human race survived for hundreds of thousands of years without smoking. Surely no one believes there is something natural about deliberately breathing in bad, cancerous fumes? The fact is that none of us had a need to smoke before we lit our first cigarette. If you are one of the unlucky ones who fell into the trap at such an early age that you cannot remember the time you didn't need to smoke, don't worry – if you had felt you were missing something, you would have remembered it! Earlier I gave my dictionary definition of brainwashing as:

'To effect a radical change in the ideas and beliefs of a person.'

It is a fact that from birth each of us is bombarded daily with so-called 'facts'. When it comes to smoking we are told that smoking relaxes us, aids concentration and helps to alleviate stress and boredom. We are also told that it is a filthy disgusting habit that will get us hooked and ruin our health and wealth if we are stupid enough to dabble with it. Ironically, the people who most emphasize the downside – our parents – are often puffing away as they do so. We believe them, but no matter how much they emphasize the evils of smoking, we are not stupid. We know that mom has to reach for her pack of cigarettes every time she gets uptight and that dad can't answer the phone without lighting up. They have said the words enough times – 'I'm gasping for a cigarette!', 'Let's get out of here, I need a cigarette!', or, in the case of an attempt to stop, 'I could murder a cigarette!' – along with showing the bad temper and frayed edges that go with a craving for nicotine.

It is wrong to say that we are being brainwashed at this stage, because our ideas and beliefs are not so much being changed as being formed. Of course this bombardment of information – both for the pros and cons of smoking – has not the slightest effect on us. At this stage we believe both sides. But because we have no need or desire to smoke before we become hooked, and can enjoy social occasions and cope with stress without the need of a cigarette, we are in the happy situation of having absolutely nothing to gain and much to lose from smoking. There is not a smoker in the entire history of the planet – indeed, there is not an alcoholic or a drug addict in the entire history of the planet – who believed they would become hooked. If they had believed this was a possibility, they would never have taken that first dose. It is only because that first cigarette tastes so bad that we are fooled into believing that we won't become hooked.

It is only after we fall into the trap that the brainwashing takes effect. In other words, prior to taking the bait we see smoking as a filthy, unhealthy and expensive habit. This first cigarette not only confirms this perception – it explodes the myth that smoking is a pleasant or enjoyable pastime. Despite this, in no time at all smoking appears to be enjoyable, relaxing and a real confidence booster. Soon we are regarding cigarettes as indispensable and it's not long before we are unable to go without them. No matter how quickly or gradually this process occurs, we seem oblivious to it. But there is no denying that our perceptions have shifted. To an optimist the bottle is half-full. The pessimist sees it as half-empty. Who has the correct perception?

IS THE BOTTLE HALF-FULL OR HALF-EMPTY?

2 *Is The Bottle Half-full Or Half-empty?*

If the bottle contains exactly 50 percent of its total capacity, both the optimist and the pessimist are correct. Both of them have a different perception of the same fact. Everyone is entitled to his own opinion, but in this book we are not concerned with opinions, only with facts. If the bottle contains either more or less than half its total capacity, both the optimist and the pessimist have a distorted perception of the true situation. When asked 'How did Allen Carr help you to stop?', some ex-smokers who have attended my clinics will reply, 'He brainwashed me into believing that I didn't need ever to smoke again.'

This reply is a cause of consternation to me. It implies that I use tactics similar to those of some cult organization which aims to control the thoughts of its members, and, more alarmingly, that it will be a simple matter for someone to reverse the process and convince that smoker that they do need to smoke again.

Hypnotherapy is part of the sessions at our clinics. After a session clients leave firmly believing that they no longer want a cigarette. But when probing questions – from both smokers and non-smokers – are put to them about what actually happens in those sessions, most clients are unable to explain and will resort to giving unenlightening replies, such as 'It's a mystery to me but it works'.

Let me assure you, we do not deal in mysticism. Nothing could be further from the truth. Ali Baba probably felt great when he could gain access to treasure by saying 'Open Sesame'. But do you really need to dabble with mysticism to open your front door? Don't you feel safer with a lock and key that only you possess? I am interested only in facts. Let me emphasize: I never use brainwashing techniques. In fact, my method – which I call Easyway – is based on counter-brainwashing.

For the purpose of this book, we need to re-define brainwashing as:

'To effectively persuade a person that certain facts and beliefs are true when in fact they are false.'

I would define counter-brainwashing as:

'A technique designed to remove the brainwashing to enable the person to see the true situation.'

Perhaps you are saying to yourself, 'Oh, no, he's surely not going to tell me that smoking is a filthy, disgusting habit that is bad for my health and costs me a fortune.'

I assure you that Easyway doesn't depend upon such tactics. You are already aware that smoking is bad for your health and this knowledge actually creates anxiety. What do smokers do when they are under stress? That's right: they reach for a cigarette.

Society generally tends to treat smokers as rather simple-minded, weak-willed, social pariahs. The majority of smokers see themselves in a similar light. After all, you are a competent person and in control of the majority of your daily affairs, yet you've lost the plot where cigarettes are concerned. This too is all part of the brainwashing. In actuality you have as much willpower – possibly more – than the next person, be they non-smoker or ex-smoker. Currently though you are using your willpower in negative polarity.

You might find some of the things I say difficult to believe. At times you might be tempted to despatch this book to the wastebin. Please don't do that. There are no horror stories in these pages. On the contrary, I have nothing but good news for you. However, we have a chicken-and-egg situation. The main factor preventing smokers from even attempting to stop is fear. This fear is real and takes many forms. The fear that in order to succeed, they must first go through an indefinite period of misery and torture. The fear that they do not have the necessary willpower to succeed. The fear of failure. Ironically, the greatest fear is the fear of success: the fear that, for the rest of our lives, meals and other social occasions will never be quite so enjoyable. After all, you've seen friends go through it and who wants to experience that misery? The fear that we won't be able to answer the telephone or cope with stress without a cigarette. The fear that, if we do manage to succeed, we'll become complaining ex-smokers and spend the rest of our lives bemoaning the fact that we daren't light another cigarette.

Let's not pretend these fears don't exist. They are both real and powerful. If you've ever attempted a 'willpower-method' of quitting, as I did on many occasions, you will know that the overall feeling is not so much that you are giving up smoking as giving up living and, moreover, giving up a coping mechanism, your support. So at this point let's accept that you have one or more of these fears. Let's also accept that it takes genuine courage to make the attempt to stop. But the fact that you have got this far means that you have already surmounted that hurdle. The beautiful truth is that those fears are all part of the brainwashing and, as such, can be removed before you actually stop smoking.

All smokers are schizophrenic. They see smoking as a sort of tug-of-war. On one side there's fear: it's killing me, costing me a fortune and controlling my life. On the other side: it's my pleasure, my companion, my crutch. Let's be honest, it's not so much that we enjoy smoking – think back to the woman in the hospital. Isn't it more that we can't enjoy life or cope with life without smoking? That side of the tug-of-war is also fear. Smoking, like all drug addiction, is a tug-of-war of fear: the fear of what the drug is doing to us, and the fear of not being able to enjoy or cope with life without it. Remember, non-smokers don't suffer from either of these fears.

One ingenuity of the trap is that the fear on one side is a fear of the future: 'OK, I might get lung cancer, then again I might be lucky.' But the moment you decide to make an attempt to stop, you are forcing yourself to face the misery of the trauma you have to go through, the fear of failure and the fear of life without smoking, today. Naturally the tendency is to postpone the evil day in the hope that you'll continue being lucky, or that you might walk under a bus, or by some miracle you will wake up one morning and never have the need or desire to smoke again.

Perhaps, like me, you have heard of smokers to whom this happened. For thirty years I prayed that it would happen to me. Get it clearly into your mind: one ingenuity of the nicotine trap is that, like all drug addiction, it is designed to keep you hooked, and that the more it adversely affects your health and purse, the more securely you appear to be hooked. It is true that a small minority of smokers do wake up one morning and lose the desire to smoke again. Invariably such smokers have reached the stage where they can no longer delude themselves that they are receiving any pleasure, or a crutch, from smoking. Sadly the vast majority who reach that stage leave it too late. Please don't let that happen to you. All our lives as smokers we promise ourselves that we'll stop tomorrow. I was lucky enough to escape before it happened to me. I can only try to imagine the self-denigration had I left it too late. If I'd actually contracted lung cancer, I'm convinced that all the brainwashing would have disappeared instantly and that my attitude would have been:

'You utter fool, you idiot! You were lucky enough to be born with a strong, healthy body. How could you be so ungrateful, or so stupid, as to spend your life poisoning your lungs with this filth? How could you have been so selfish to be insensitive to the anguish you were causing to the people that loved you? You think of yourself as a rational, intelligent human being. How can you have been so stupid and weak to bring this on yourself?'

Perhaps you still believe that I'm appealing to your rationality. Not so; I'm simply trying to imagine what my thoughts would have been at the time. The point is that no smoker would have such thoughts unless and until they had left it too late. I'm simply trying to point out the ingenuity of the trap. As I have said, this is the chicken-and-egg situation. The beautiful truth is that both sets of fears are simply part of the brainwashing and as such can be removed before you finish the book. So be prepared in advance. Accept, indeed expect, that there might be times when you are tempted not to complete the book, or to read it oh so slowly, diverting yourself from it by finding more pressing things to do, such as running the house, feeding the children and having a career.

We all accept that life is a gamble. In our struggle to enjoy and cope with life, we can never be sure that one particular course of action will be to our benefit or detriment. But how many times in our lives are we in the position of having absolutely nothing to lose and everything to gain from a decision we make? You are in that enviable position now. Do you think I exaggerate? Not so. I want you to promise me, and, more importantly, to promise yourself, that you will complete the book. Be aware that the trap is designed to imprison you for life. Don't allow yourself to be fooled by it. If you complete the book:

YOU HAVE ABSOLUTELY NOTHING TO LOSE!

If you want to, you can continue to smoke. In fact, you will feel better. Instead of feeling stupid and guilty, you will be able to say to your family and friends: 'I did my best. I read it through and through and still I can't stop!' You will have done all that I, or anyone else, could ask of you, and you will be able to continue smoking with a completely clear conscience. Get it clearly into your mind: you have absolutely nothing to lose. So, there is no need to feel gloomy as you continue reading. I promise you that I have nothing but good news for you. You don't even have to stop or cut down while you are reading the book. On the contrary. This might sound stupid advice, but unless you have decided that you have already smoked your final cigarette, it will actually help you not to attempt to stop or even to cut down before you finish the book. However, don't use this as an excuse to read one line a day. If you have already smoked what you hope will be your last cigarette, finish the book as quickly as you can.

When I refer to cigarette smoking, as I do throughout the book, take this to mean any form of smoking, from pipes and cigars to roll-ups, indeed any form of taking nicotine, including snuff, chewing gum, patches or nasal sprays.

Don't let the fact that you have absolutely nothing to lose blinker you to the powerful gains you will make through Easyway. There is far more to gain than simply keeping more cash in your pocket or smelling sweeter. Among the compliments I receive from those who discover their freedom through the Easyway method is:

'Thank you for giving me my life.'

Another is:

'My life began when I stopped smoking.'

I receive letters from heavy, long-term smokers, as I was, male and female, as well as from younger people. When we are slaves to nicotine we cannot block the mind to the risks we are running. Like you, no doubt, I'd had so many failed attempts that I was finding it increasingly difficult even to kid myself that I would stop before IT happened. I was waiting, expecting and resigned to the fact that smoking would kill me some day. Ironically, it didn't bother me unduly. I'd sunk so low that death didn't appear to be such a bad option. Of course, it hadn't occurred to me – nor will it have to you – that smoking was responsible for reducing me to such a state. Oh, I knew it was making me breathless, but I'd attributed my lack of energy and permanent feeling of tiredness to getting older and trying to do too much. What never occurred to me was the effect it was having on me psychologically. On the contrary, I genuinely believed that smoking gave me courage and confidence. After all, we all know that having a cappuccino in a café without a cigarette as an accompaniment is like being naked, and trying to break the ice at a party without cigarettes leaves us feeling even more exposed. I knew I would never be able to concentrate properly without smoking. How could you get away from the madding crowd without your ciggy break? In fact, that packet of cigarettes was not only my best friend but my strength. Without it I was a jellyfish, lacking the capacity or desire to enjoy life, or cope with it.

When the fog is lifted from your eyes, it is like awakening from a permanent nightmare. I was released from a black and white world of fear and depression into a sunshine, technicolor world of energy, confidence and control. For nearly a third of a century I'd forgotten the sensation of just feeling great to be alive. Like most smokers, I got hooked in my teens and associated my loss of joy of living with a combination of advancing age and the responsibilities of adulthood. When I stopped, I expected to be healthier and wealthier, and believed that these would be the greatest benefits. In fact, they were superseded by several others, including:

1. The replacement of self-despising with self-respect.

2. The replacement of feeling insecure with unconditional confidence.

3. The removal of that ever-increasing black shadow, which, no matter how we try to block our minds to it, all drug addicts suffer from the moment they take the second dose. From that point on, either consciously or sub-consciously, we spend the rest of our lives lying to ourselves. Initially we tell ourselves that we won't get hooked. When eventually it dawns on us that we are already dangling from that hook, we promise ourselves that we will stop – but not today, tomorrow. Always it's tomorrow. I'll explain later why tomorrow never comes.

4. The ending of the slavery. We are so obsessed with resisting the efforts of society, including ourselves, to force us to stop, it never dawns on us that we get no particular pleasure from smoking when we are actually doing it. In fact, we take it for granted. This is why we think the vast majority of cigarettes we smoke are just habitual. Many smokers will say their favourite

cigarette is the one they have after a meal. Let's look at this assertion. Why should the same cigarette out of the same packet taste any different from the others? In truth, it can't. There's no difference in its contents. It's not so much that smokers particularly enjoy a cigarette after a meal, but that an otherwise enjoyable occasion is actually made miserable if they aren't allowed to smoke. The lives of non-smokers aren't dominated in this way. What sort of pleasure can this be? On the rare occasions when we face up to the facts about smoking, we wish we had never started. Cigarettes only become precious to us when we aren't allowed to smoke. Can you think of any pastime, other than drug addiction, that works in this way? Only when you aren't allowed to do it, you wish you could, and when you are allowed to, you wish you didn't have to?

But the sum total of the benefits of stopping smoking is greater than the individual gains we've been discussing. Before I became a non-smoker, I used to wake up each morning feeling tired and lethargic; this after ten hours' sleep. Then I would have to force myself out of bed to face the trials and tribulations of the day. Now in my seventies, I wake up feeling fully rested, energetic and looking forward to what lies ahead. That's what people mean when they say:

'My life began when I stopped smoking.'

I was sent an exceptionally inspiring letter by a young lady called Debbie Sekula:

'I laughed to myself about how I had become so desperate to stop smoking I was resorting to a book. It seemed illogical and pathetic. It made no sense that scientifically devised methods of quitting smoking would fail and a book would succeed.'

Like so many areas in life, when it comes to stopping smoking often we seek out so-called expert views to assure ourselves that we are taking the best course of action in order to succeed. In the world of the nicotine addict, though, everything we think we know about the trap and how we are supposed to get out of it is usually the complete opposite of the reality.

Strange as it may seem, this book will change the way you perceive cigarettes, not just when you finish reading it but for the rest of your life. The thing that excites me most is the fact that it is simply information that provides you with the mental tools you need to understand how to escape. Knowledge is power: without it you feel at a loss, with it you feel like a winner. Debbie's words say it all:

'It was then that I was overcome with the knowledge that I had a smile on my face that I could not get rid of. As I turned the final page of your book that Sunday afternoon, I knew that I would never smoke again. I knew that for once and for all, I was cured.

'It was such an amazing feeling. I can't explain it, but I'm sure you know the feeling I mean…

'I am now into my second week. I am still just as happy and excited, if not more so, as I was when I finished your book. I am experiencing a new world of smells, taste, energy. I can't believe how great I feel!

'My life at the moment is one big miracle. Everything feels new and fantastic. You opened the door for me to walk through, and I can't thank you enough.

'You talk about a revelation that can happen any time over three weeks or so. With me it was seconds! I don't even think about smoking any more.

'I will close by saying Thank You.

'I hope to get the opportunity to thank you in person some day, but in lieu of that opportunity, THANK YOU SO MUCH FOR TEACHING ME HOW TO LIVE!

'With all my Love and Best Wishes to you and your obviously Loving family.

Debbie Sekula.'

I've lost count of the thousands of similar letters I've received over the years. You might remember that earlier, in relation to my own quitting, I referred to:

'When the miracle happened it was like awakening from a permanent nightmare.'

In her letter Debbie comments, 'My life at the moment is one big miracle.' Another phrase that appears regularly in such letters is: 'It was like magic', or something similar. Let's take a closer look at these twins:

MIRACLE OR MAGIC?

3 *Miracle Or Magic?*

In truth, it was neither miracle nor magic; it just seemed like it at the time. Many years later it still does. I'd been a chain-smoker for nearly a third of a century. It wasn't so much that I enjoyed smoking but that I didn't seem able to function without it. I'd had umpteen failed attempts to stop, once even surviving six months without cigarettes. But I never felt like a non-smoker. I even believed – no doubt as you currently believe – that there were different types of smoker. There were, for example, social smokers – people who were just going through the motions. You only have to look at them to see they aren't enjoying it. They really don't look like real smokers. They want to feel part of the crowd and so only smoke on social occasions. They always look uncomfortable, never inhale, keep forgetting to flick the ash and as a rule only smoke 'freemans', usually yours.

Then there is the type that every 'heavy' smoker envied – the casual smoker who apparently enjoyed each cigarette immensely, could inhale deeply without coughing, had several smoking affectations and really looked the part. Yet, incredibly, they only ever seemed to need or desire about five cigarettes a day. The predominant group seemed to be the habitual smoker, the type I referred to previously, who only enjoyed two of the twenty they smoked each day. They appeared not to derive any particular pleasure from smoking, seemed to have drifted into the habit and claimed they would stop if it began to affect their health. Then there was my group – the real smokers. Deep down inside these people knew they were completely dependent on tobacco and couldn't enjoy life, concentrate or handle stress without a cigarette. The term 'smokaholic' hadn't yet been coined. But, just as many alcoholics believe they have a different chemical make-up to normal drinkers, so I believed there must be a difference in the chemical make-up of smokers like me and that of normal smokers. I was also convinced that had I been able to conjure up sufficient willpower to stop, no matter how long I lasted, I would always be a smoker who wasn't allowed to smoke.

Then it happened, as if a thick and ever-present veil had been lifted from my eyes: I could see smoking without the brainwashing. Even before I'd put out my final cigarette, I knew I was already a non-smoker. I knew for certain that I would never, ever have a need or desire to smoke again. What I didn't understand immediately was why it was so easy. Why didn't I have the terrible withdrawal symptoms I'd suffered previously when attempting to stop? I had no withdrawal symptoms whatsoever and actually enjoyed the entire process of quitting.

At this stage, you may have several questions you'd like answered. I've no doubt the first one is: 'Can you tell me what happened to you and how can you make it happen to me?'

How can I make it happen to you? I can't. But you are, in fact, already doing it by yourself. All you have to do is complete the book with an open mind. This means you shouldn't meekly accept everything that I tell you. On the contrary, it is essential to question everything I tell you, and everything that society has brainwashed you to believe. By opening your mind to challenge your perception of cigarettes, and what you have been conditioned to think about smoking, you will be able to make the informed choices that will become available to you later in the book.

The 'why' is happening now as you read, and it will continue for the whole of this book. You might be thinking that if you had reached the same stage of degradation as me, you too would have stopped without difficulty. Remember, that didn't stop me. I was expecting to die and still I couldn't stop. You probably know people who are dying prematurely as a result of contracting a smoking-related disease and yet haven't stopped. If you were in their position neither would you. Visiting sick and dying relatives or friends makes us feel bad, but in such a situation we rely on those cigarettes even more, despite the shame and guilt. You have only to look outside the main door of any hospital to know this is true.

Perhaps my mentioning different types of smokers has made you wonder if you belong to a type that Easyway doesn't work for. I used to wonder, too, before I understood the nicotine trap. Imagine for a moment smoking as a self-imposed prison. Every lock requires a key to open it easily. Easyway is the key that will enable any smoker to escape immediately from the nicotine trap. There are different categories of smokers, but just as identical twins are not completely identical, so every individual smoker is unique.

I hope you are already aware of my reputation and are reading this book because of a recommendation from an 'escapee'. Indeed you might even have read one or more of my previous books or attended one of my centres. If so, you might also have heard of smokers who tried Easyway, but did not succeed. Why did they not succeed?

I can only give them the key, I can no more force them to use it than I could force you to get on a bus if you didn't want to! Now I've probably set you worrying that part of your brain doesn't want you to use that key.

After all, even if you hate being a smoker with all your heart and cannot think of a single aspect in its favour, accept that it's only you who lights the cigarette. Whether you understand it or not, there is something in your brain that makes you contradict your rational thoughts, otherwise you would already be a non-smoker. At this stage, don't worry about it. Easyway will remove the doubt. Remember that you have absolutely nothing to lose. Finish the book first, then decide if you want to stop. By the end of the book, you'll be free, like Debbie.

At this point your view of smoking will be blurred, like one of those 3D pictures, and while you don't have the correct approach it will remain so. The moment you look at the situation from a re-evaluated standpoint the image will become crystal clear.

There are several reasons why I've chosen to include Debbie's letter. Let's look again at some of the points she made:

'I laughed to myself about how I had become so desperate to stop smoking that I was resorting to reading a book! The thought was so pathetic and illogical to me. It made no sense that scientifically devised methods of quitting smoking would fail and that a book would succeed.'

Debbie was obviously very sceptical about Easyway, as are all smokers in the beginning. Even so, she did finish the book and it's quite obvious that she did succeed. She clearly understood the 'why'. But perhaps you will question whether she had actually succeeded in the long term. After all, she was only in her second week at the time of writing and received opinion tells us it takes far longer than that.

This is yet another example of the ludicrous conditioning we have been subjected to. The 'experts' at ASH judge success as having gone a year without smoking a cigarette. Does that sound scientific to you? Why a year? On what scientific evidence is this time-scale based? If it were true, no one would get hooked again who had managed to stop for a year! Yet there are countless cases of smokers who have stopped for several years and got hooked again. In fact, our centres are often attended by smokers who have stopped by using willpower and have managed to abstain for several years. So why do they need to attend our centres?

Because they still feel vulnerable and are still having to use willpower to resist temptation. At the centres we remove this need to 'resist the temptation'. One of the reasons I don't like being referred to as a guru is that it implies that Easyway is based on mystical or spiritual powers. True, it might seem like a miracle or magic, but it is based on science, common sense and fact. Just as I knew I was free before I put out my final cigarette, so did Debbie. She didn't have to wait until the second week:

'To be quite honest, my doubts ran away about halfway through your book. It was then that I was overcome with the knowledge that I had a smile on my face which I could not get rid of! As I turned the final page of your book that Sunday afternoon, I knew that I would never smoke again! I knew that for once and for all, I was cured.'

Incidentally, this is quite common at our centres. During the middle of the therapy, a client might say something like:

'You needn't say another word. I know I shall never smoke again.'

Even so we ensure that the client completes the therapy. From feedback I have learned that many smokers enjoy this same experience before they have completed the book. Hopefully this will happen to you. If it does, you must still complete the book. It's no good just obtaining the state of euphoria that Debbie so accurately describes. We must ensure that you retain it so that you are never tempted to smoke again.

This brings me to a matter I loathe to address but nevertheless feel duty bound to. Perhaps you have heard of smokers who successfully used Easyway for several weeks or even years, only to fall into the trap again. They seem to have lost the euphoria. Unfortunately, this can happen. But if, for argument's sake, Debbie were to fall into the trap again after three months, a doctor (the 'expert') might knowingly shake his head and say sagely:

'There you see! She wasn't really cured. You can't regard a smoker as cured until they have abstained for at least a year!'

This same 'expert' will conveniently overlook the fact that, on the same basis, you cannot regard smokers as cured after they have abstained for a year. The 'expert's' measure of success also fails completely to consider the mental state of the ex-smoker at any stage during the period of abstinence, as if it were irrelevant. On this evidence I define such 'experts' as people who purport to be but aren't.

To 'give up' smoking is by far the most popular New Year resolution. I know of several cases where smokers manage to survive the whole year without a cigarette and then declare: 'EUREKA! I've kicked it!' Believing they are now safe, they actually celebrate by having just one cigarette. Before they know it, they are back in the trap. You may have experienced this yourself. In such cases it is correct to say that those smokers, far from succeeding because they abstained for a year, failed because they stopped for a year. The doctor will certainly tend to overlook the fact that with a 'willpower' method the chances of success are less than 10 percent. At our centres we refund a client's fee if they fail to stop for at least three months.

Coincidentally, the percentage is the same, but for the opposite reason – worldwide fewer than 10 percent of our clients find it necessary to claim a refund and more than 80 percent of our clients come to us as a direct result of recommendation.

You might find these figures difficult to accept. Indeed, we have been criticized for citing them, but true they are. Bear in mind that I'm not like ASH or QUIT, powerful institutions receiving enormous sponsorship or charitable funds. Nor do I have the finances of the international drug conglomerates which, every few years, launch massive TV campaigns to advertise their latest pill or patch. By the end of the book you will understand exactly why these products are just gimmicks.

I'm just a lone individual who never advertises. Yet my first book, *The Easy Way to Stop Smoking*, has been a bestseller every year since its first publication in 1985. It is now printed in over 40 languages and was a No. 1 bestseller in Germany for a year and reached No. 2 in Holland.

We now have over 150 centres distributed in every continent with the exception of Antarctica. Any applicants? Every Easyway therapist is an ex-smoker who themselves stopped with the help of the method and recognized its unique effectiveness. Note that Debbie lives on the other side of the world and that just as you are reading this book because you have heard of my reputation so did she and her boyfriend. Why then throughout the world is Allen Carr the equivalent in terms of stopping smoking as Lionel Messi is to football?

There is one reason and one reason alone: Easyway works.

However, I digress. I have possibly distracted you from a more important question that you should be asking yourself at this moment. If you can't rely on the 'experts' to define what is getting free,

HOW CAN YOU EVER KNOW
WHEN YOU ARE CURED?

4 *How Can You Ever Know When You Are Cured?*

Before I discovered Easyway I firmly believed that you could never know for sure. The 'experts' reinforced that notion for me. Let's take a look at a typical attempt to stop smoking using a 'willpower' method.

I define a 'willpower' method as any method other than Easyway. It would include Zyban or NRT (Nicotine Replacement Therapy, such as patches, gum or nasal sprays). Typically with this method you start off with a feeling of doom and gloom yet hoping that you might succeed if you can survive the misery and craving long enough. But how long do you have to wait? Who knows? We've already established that even abstinence for a whole year is not proof against failure.

Not only is this a miserable and frightening situation, but you are in the ludicrous situation of actually waiting for nothing to happen. A typical platitude voiced by the 'experts' is: 'Remember, the longer you can last out the misery, the greater your chances of success.'

This is designed to boost your willpower to enable you to continue holding out. The problem is that it works. And it might seem like good positive advice, unless and until you analyse it.

What this little snippet actually means is: if I can survive ten years without a cigarette, my chances of success are greater than if I give in after an hour. Brilliant! I never would have worked that out for myself. In practice, if you follow such advice, you simply prolong the misery. This is what I meant when I talked about using willpower in negative polarity. The longer you hold out the longer the torture. Let's put it in different terms: a child wants a toy and you take it away. What happens? The child with no willpower will get over the conflict quickly and that will be the end of the matter. But the child with tremendous willpower will go on and on, sometimes into adulthood, dragging up the incident, usually when the mind and tongue are loosened by alcohol. Similarly the complaining stopper will, twenty years after having stopped smoking, bemoan the absence of nicotine when drunk or confronted by a stressful situation.

Let me describe my final attempt using 'willpower'. I had survived a full six months without so much as a puff of a cigarette or cigar. People who had stopped successfully by using willpower had led me to believe that it's tough to begin with but, provided you can hang on, gradually it gets easier and eventually the cravings become so few and far between they don't bother you. In truth, to begin with, I didn't find it so bad. This was probably because I knew I hadn't long to live if I didn't stop and was very determined to succeed. The problem was – as you know from your own experience – that instead of the misery and craving gradually getting easier, it just got worse and worse. After six months I was a nervous wreck, incapable of completing any task that involved even the slightest use of the grey matter. And I gave in. I cried like a baby, partly because I felt so low, partly because I'd failed to achieve something that I'd set out to achieve, partly because I knew that I could never be free. However, I cried mainly because I doubted that if I could have lasted out another day, week or month I might have succeeded. I despised myself for giving in. I'm sure you recognize yourself in this scene to some extent.

Now that I understand smoking completely (as you are starting to), I realize that no matter how long I had held out, I had no more chance of succeeding than I would have of skiing up the Matterhorn. I was just using my willpower to prolong the misery. Because I believed that I couldn't enjoy life, or concentrate, or handle stress without smoking before I put out what I hoped would be my final cigarette, the misery I was going through, far from removing that belief, was simply magnifying it. It didn't seem so at the time, but I took what was a perfectly rational decision, based on the information I had and the beliefs I held. I decided, 'If this is life without nicotine, I'm opting for the shorter, but sweeter life of the smoker.' (In case you are thinking of doing the same, it's true that the smoker's life is shorter, but in no way can it be described as sweeter. I will expand on this later.)

Bear in mind that I went through all that misery only because I fell into the trap and not because I was trying to escape from it. Non-smokers never have to suffer such tortures. I promise you, complete the book, follow my advice, and you'll soon know what real pleasure is.

Perhaps you are wondering how on earth any smoker manages to escape using 'willpower'. I could explain, but both my time and yours is better spent concentrating on how to make the escape easy and enjoyable. Nevertheless some do eventually succeed. It's clear that they can only speculate how long it will take and most are still taking it one day at a time, like a recovering alcoholic as a work colleague put it. But there is another major flaw with the willpower method; we have been taught that you can never be free.

It is important that you give the following question considerable thought: When do you know you are cured? When you have come up with what you believe to be the correct answer, compare it with the typical answers we receive from clients at our centres:

'When I can go a whole day (week etc.) without smoking.'

You might remember Debbie's comment: 'any other attempt in the past had become a failure in a matter of hours.' However, this does help to illustrate the fear that smoking creates. Occasionally you meet long-term smokers who claim to enjoy smoking so much that they've never had the desire to stop. I used to believe them. The truth is that they are too frightened even to try. This is something else you will soon learn: that no matter how honest they are in other matters, all smokers lie, even to themselves – they have to! Unfortunately, the fact that a smoker hasn't managed to abstain for even a day previously is no guarantee that once they do manage to abstain they'll be free.

'When I've gone a year without a cigarette.'

This is a very common belief, which we have already addressed. But can you imagine the terror such a statement has on the previous group? No wonder we put off the evil day.

'When I can go to a party and enjoy it.'

That's more like it, but how do they know they'll enjoy the next party?

'When I feel like a non-smoker.'

I used to believe that smokers felt different from non-smokers. But non-smokers don't feel like non-smokers, any more than non-heroin addicts feel like non-heroin addicts. That feeling like a smoker is really a feeling that you won't be able to enjoy life or cope without cigarettes. It's not a very pleasant feeling and you'll soon be delighted to be rid of it.

'When I can concentrate without a cigarette.'

This was the one that kept me hooked. If you believe cigarettes help you to concentrate, no matter how long you survive without one, whenever you have a mental block, as everybody does, you'll just sit there bemoaning the fact that you can't have a cigarette, thereby guaranteeing that you won't be able to concentrate.

'I don't know.'

Doesn't sound too encouraging, but at least it's honest and the people who respond in this way have deduced that answers 1 to 5 are inaccurate.

'Never!'

I used to believe that. I'm so pleased I was wrong.

'When I stop thinking about smoking.'

I quote Debbie again:

'I don't even think about smoking any more.'

This is a common theme of the letters I receive, so is it the missing slate? Is it the key to Easyway? After all, one cannot deny that Debbie was reasonably happy to be a non-smoker:

'Reading your book, and taking that chance, well, that was the best and most incredible decision I have ever made. ... I had a smile on my face which I could not get rid of! ... I am still just as happy and excited, if not more so, as I was when I finished your book! ... I am experiencing a new world of smells, taste energy!! ... I can't believe how great I feel! ... I actually glow! ... My life at the moment is one big miracle ... Everything feels new and fantastic ... I'm gushing! See how excited I am ... It was such an amazing feeling!! I can't explain it, but I'm sure you know the feeling I mean! You opened the door for me to walk through, and I can't thank you enough! You, however, have made an impact on my life so huge that I can not begin to express the way I feel about you and your method.'

Yes, Debbie, even after so many years of freedom, I well remember that feeling. I think you'll agree with me that she expressed both her feelings and her thanks more than capably.

I'm often asked: 'How does Easyway work?'

Me: 'Smokers arrive at our centres in various stages of panic, believing that they have to go through an indefinite period of misery and that, even if they are lucky enough to succeed, social occasions will never be quite so enjoyable and that they'll be less capable of handling stress. Over 90 percent of them leave four hours later already happy non-smokers.'

'What on earth do you say to them?'

Me: 'Have you four hours to spare?'

They think I'm being evasive, and perhaps you are coming to the same conclusion. I assure you that I am not. Clearly Debbie took great care in formulating her letter. She has been very articulate in expressing her euphoria and generous in giving me all the credit:

'You opened the door for me to walk through.'

But she didn't experience the euphoria until after she'd walked through that 'door'. With the exception of one possible clue, what she doesn't do is to explain how Easyway enabled someone who had only managed to abstain for a few hours previously to stop so easily. True, she listed certain benefits she had received, but that wasn't the clue. She was fully aware of those benefits before she read the book. All smokers know they'll receive powerful benefits if they can manage to stop. Why else would you be trying to do it? So what is the clue? Is it, 'I don't even think about smoking any more.'?

No, this is another piece of advice from the 'experts', and one that more than any other makes the 'willpower' method such a nightmare. It sounds logical:

Expert: 'Try to distract your mind. Avoid situations that remind you of smoking.'

You: 'Brilliant! Why didn't I think of that?'

Think on –

You: 'Of course my partner smokes, but a split could be arranged. And as for my smoking friends, I'll just boycott them. After all, I can soon make new ones. Wait a minute, though, people smoke in restaurants and bars or at social clubs, places I'm likely to go to make new friends.

Oh well, I'll have to avoid them as well. In fact, I'll only ever be able to socialize if there's not a single smoker present. Hang on a minute, though: I may never be able to go out again, let alone socialize, because cigarettes are available at every shopping outlet on the planet. And then there's my job – people smoke at work. I'll have to give it up.'

Expert: 'Come, come, you're taking this too far and exaggerating the situation. You need only avoid smokers until you have succeeded.'

You: 'And how long will that be?'

Here comes the rub – the 'experts' advise that it'll be at least a year – maybe.

You: 'That's helpful! What do you suggest I do in the meantime? Sit alone in a room playing patience?'

It's little wonder that so few smokers manage to succeed when using 'willpower' methods.

Have you ever found you couldn't sleep at night because you had a problem on your mind? Did counting sheep distract you? Or did you find that no matter how much you tried to distract yourself the problem would keep going round and round in your head? Did you also find that your lack of sleep became an additional problem and that the more you worried the more you ensured that you didn't get to sleep? And I'll warrant that when you did finally drop off into a deep, restful slumber, within five minutes that alarm clock brought you out of it.

Smoking takes up whole lives. When she wrote to me Debbie hadn't stopped thinking about smoking. Her entire letter was devoted solely to the subject of smoking. I spend most of my life thinking about smoking.

For the first few hours, days, weeks or even months, smokers who are attempting to 'give up' with the use of willpower are also obsessed with the subject of smoking. But the difference is that they are thinking: 'When will this misery end? Will I ever stop craving cigarettes?' When Debbie and I think about smoking, we are thinking: 'Isn't it great? I'm free! I haven't the slightest need or desire to light up.'

So is that the key? Is it really as simple as that? From this moment, whenever I am tempted to light up, instead of doing so, all I have to say to myself is: 'Isn't it great!? I'm free! I haven't the slightest need or desire to light up.' Would that really work? It might for a few days, but don't waste your time trying it. The point is, you have to know it's true. It's no good just saying it, You must understand and believe it.

Whether they have the courage to admit it or not, all smokers believe themselves to be stupid, weak-willed people. I'm frequently cornered at social functions by smokers who want to convince me of the pleasure and crutch they get from smoking. If you think they do this simply to resist my attempts to convert them, you would be wrong. When you have spent ten hours a day, seven days a week doing just that, the one conversation you try to avoid is about smoking. In any event, I soon learned that you have more chance of persuading a giant clam to open up than persuading smokers to 'give up' before they have decided to. I listen patiently, thinking 'I enjoy eating peas but I don't feel the need to justify it to someone who doesn't'. When my patience is exhausted, I simply ask the person if they encourage their children or grandchildren to smoke. They then spend the remainder of the evening telling me how pleased they are that their offspring have heeded their advice and don't smoke, or how disappointed they are that they do, in spite of all their advice and pleading. When I point out that I can't understand why, if they get so much pleasure from smoking, and it is such a crutch for them, they don't encourage their offspring to smoke, they stare at me as if I am the one who is confused.

As I will explain later, heavy smokers are often particularly intelligent and strong-willed. But most smokers believe themselves to be stupid because they smoke, and a few believe the reverse: that they smoke because they are stupid. Neither statement is true. Even the most intelligent people occasionally do stupid things.

Both intelligent and less intelligent people might accidentally fall off a roof or step under a bus, but the only reason they would do that deliberately would be to commit suicide. Nobody continues to smoke accidentally, whether they have an incredibly high IQ or severe learning difficulties. The vast majority of cigarettes we smoke are smoked subconsciously. Even the ritual of reaching for the packet and lighting up is usually performed subconsciously. However, when we run out, the act of buying or sponging more cigarettes is a deliberate and conscious act.

Get it clearly into your mind: there is a reason for every cigarette that you smoke, and that reason isn't because you are either weak-willed or stupid. You may think you know what the true reason is. I assure you that you don't, because if you did, you would have no reason to be reading this book. You would already be a happy non-smoker and would remain one for the rest of your life.

The important point is the effect. You started this book feeling down, humble and full of dread, but soon you will feel elated. And stop worrying about how Easyway works. Debbie started off not only sceptical but actually scoffing at the notion that a book could help her to stop. What you cannot deny is that when she finished that book she was euphoric, and even more so over a week later. Literally millions of smokers have also found it easy to stop smoking by using Easyway. Now let me tell you about:

MY CLAIM

5 My Claim

I not only refer to my method as Easyway, but as the only way to stop smoking. Because of this, I have been accused of being both stupid and arrogant. When I say, 'the only way', I don't mean that there aren't other methods. On the contrary, I've already referred to them repeatedly, and identified them all as 'willpower' methods. I refer to Easyway as 'the only way' because it is more effective than any other method. All other methods actually make it more difficult for you to stop. Let me explain.

The current logic of health professionals with regard to smoking is the equivalent of suggesting to someone who can't swim to try substituting lead arm bands for water wings or tying their legs together. These professionals believe they are acting in the best interests of their patients, but it doesn't take much thinking to come to the conclusion that this is not the case. They could only be said to be acting in this way if they didn't know about the best option.

Let's stick to the swimming analogy to prove my point. What advice would you give to someone who wants to learn to swim? You might suggest that they start with breast stroke, crawl, back stroke, or perhaps you would get them to try floating or treading water? It wouldn't surprise me to learn that one group of people finds one method easier, while another group favours a different approach. So why shouldn't the same maxim apply to stopping smoking? However, if I were to ask if you would advise your novice to swap water wings for lead arm bands or tied legs, you would not hesitate to refute the idea, would you? Would any swimming instructor be stupid enough to put either option to any pupil?

Imagine that you knew of a method that would enable you to stop smoking

- EASILY, PAINLESSLY AND IMMEDIATELY

- WITHOUT SUFFERING FROM WITHDRAWAL SYMPTOMS

- WITHOUT REQUIRING YOU TO USE WILLPOWER

- WITHOUT REQUIRING YOU TO TAKE PILLS, AIDS OR GIMMICKS OR TO SUFFER AN INITIAL PERIOD OF MISERY

- AND THAT ENABLED YOU TO ENJOY SOCIAL OCCASIONS MORE.

- IMAGINE THAT YOU KNEW OF A METHOD THAT LEFT YOU BETTER EQUIPPED TO HANDLE STRESS

- YOU'LL BE: LESS NERVOUS AND TENSE

- MORE CONFIDENT AND COURAGEOUS

- BETTER ABLE TO CONCENTRATE

- NEVER, EVER CRAVING ANOTHER CIGARETTE – ALL WITHOUT COSTING YOU EXTRA KILOS.

What would you say to such a proposition?

According to the experts, such a method would be too good to be true. How could it exist? For one thing, it would have the opposite effect of those willpower methods, and make stopping easy. But just assume for a moment that such a method did exist, and that it had the added bonus of allowing you to continue to smoke while you learned how to apply it. Would you need any other method?

If you used this method and found that it worked exactly as I have stated, and understood it sufficiently to know that it would be equally effective for all smokers who decided they wanted to stop, would you recommend another system that actually made it harder to stop? If you did, wouldn't that be like advising the trainee swimmer to wear lead arm bands instead of water wings?

I have good news for you. The method I described above does exist. I call it Easyway, and you are already starting to use it.

But if my claim is true, shouldn't the medical profession know about it? And do you not agree that if they recommend any other method they are actually making it harder for their patients to stop?

We have been brainwashed to believe that stopping smoking is incredibly difficult.

Yet thousands of smokers have given up overnight without any hassle whatsoever, without seeking the help of Allen Carr or any other person, aid or gimmick. You probably know or have heard of such people. Yet they don't experience the same feeling of euphoria that Debbie and I, and the majority of ex-smokers who use Easyway, describe. Remarkably, though, they find stopping smoking relatively easy.

The difference between those smokers and me is that they don't know why they found it so easy. They try to analyse the reasons and are often more than happy to pass on their 'expertise' to help other smokers to stop. Before I discovered Easyway, I tried such methods. Some of them actually worked, but only for short periods. I've heard other people's stories about these methods at my centres. Sometimes at group sessions a client will begin recommending their 'method' to the other participants. I ask them why they are attending the centre if their method made it so easy:

'I assure you it was! I had no desire to smoke for several years, but then I was stupid. I had just one cigarette. I didn't even need it … '

You don't need me to tell you the rest. I then ask them why they didn't just use their method again? The reply is always: 'I did, but it didn't work this time.'

There can be no doubt that society generally, including people who have never smoked, believes it is very difficult to stop. There are also many smokers who believe, as I once did, that for some smokers it is impossible. But just ponder this belief for a moment. Why should it be difficult to stop, let alone impossible? We've already established that no one but ourselves forces us to light up. So if you decide that you never want to smoke again, why should it be difficult to do just that? There is absolutely nothing else you need to do. It's simplicity itself – you are already a non-smoker!

Surely it can't be as simple as that? Everyone knows that smoking is a habit and that habits are difficult to break. This is another old chestnut that the 'experts' use to show off their knowledge. A cursory examination discloses that all these 'experts' are revealing is their lack of understanding. In fact, both statements are misleading: we don't smoke out of habit; and even if we did, it would be ridiculously easy to break. So, here and now, let's reject the myth that we smoke out of habit.

What is a habit? It's a repeated pattern of behaviour. Get rid of the repetition and there's no habit. What's of interest here is the cause of the repetition. Let's use a couple of examples to clarify the situation.

For most of my life, I've driven on the left-hand side of the road. I don't do this just because I got into the habit of doing it. When I drive in countries where the rule is to drive on the right, I break that habit easily and immediately, for obvious reasons. Do you see the point? Habit never explains why we repeat behaviour. To find it easy to break a habit, you need to remove the cause of the habitual behaviour. Fortunately, I have never been a nail-biter, but I know that people who do bite their fingernails can find it very difficult to break the habit, even those who would dearly love to do so. They find it difficult because they don't know the true reason why they bite their nails, or, if they do know it, don't know how to remove that reason.

However, let us assume for the moment that the only reason we continue to smoke is because we have got into the habit of smoking. If that were true, why on earth would the habit be difficult to break? It would be simplicity itself: just don't light another cigarette. You don't even have to do anything!

The other reason the 'experts' give to explain why 'giving up' is difficult is: the terrible physical withdrawal symptoms. This is another myth and just as easy to explode. I must admit that even when I'd put out my final cigarette and knew I would never smoke again, I was still expecting to have to endure terrible physical withdrawal symptoms. I didn't have any. But how could I have avoided them? After all, I hadn't used NRT. It wasn't until I looked back at my previous 'willpower' attempts and tried to remember what happened that it dawned on me that I hadn't experienced physical pain then either.

At our centres the majority of clients require just one four-hour session. Occasionally, a client will ring up and a conversation similar to the following will ensue:

Client: 'You told me there would be no physical pain, but I'm going through torture.'

Me: 'Where does it hurt?'

Client: 'It's like flu'.

Me: 'And your doctor has told you it's withdrawal from nicotine?'

Client: 'I haven't consulted my doctor and I know it's not flu.'

Me: 'Describe the symptoms.'

Client: 'I keep breaking out in sweats!'

Me: 'So does Mary Peters every time she runs, but it doesn't seem to bother her unduly.'

Client: 'But I can't sleep at night.'

Me: 'Everybody has times when they can't sleep.'

C: 'But I can't concentrate either!'

Me: 'I don't doubt what you are saying, but none of the symptoms you have described add up to physical pain.'

The stupid thing is that, if, in order to stop, all we had to do was suffer a bout of flu for a few days, we would jump at the opportunity. When we do succumb to flu, we might feel we are dying, but we don't get all tearful and anxious. We can handle it and take it on the chin. Don't misunderstand me; I wasn't trying to underplay the torture that smoker was going through, either to her or to you. That torture is real; remember I once went through it for six months. What I am trying to get across to both her and you is that there was no physical pain. Smokers can sleep soundly throughout the night without smoking. They've gone eight hours without a cigarette. They don't wake up pulling their hair out. In fact, nowadays the vast majority of smokers get out of bed before they light up. Most don't smoke in the bedroom. Many will have tea, coffee or even breakfast first. Some will leave the house before they light up and others will wait until they get to work. Even they are not screaming in agony or climbing up the wall. But once they get to work and are about to light up, if you were to snatch the cigarette out of their mouth and grab the packet, they would break your arm!

Imagine you were going to your doctor with the symptoms you experience when that 'I want a cigarette' feeling comes on. How would you describe this sensation or pinpoint its location? Try to do this when you haven't had a cigarette for the last thirty minutes and you start to get that feeling.

When the sensation occurs, deliberately stop yourself lighting up, then try to pinpoint exactly where it hurts.

Imagine your body is like a map not dissimilar to the type used by acupuncturists. Can you even remotely fix a point where the sensation occurs? The truth is that you cannot. What you experience is just a growing feeling of unrest and imbalance which all the time you know you can get rid of by lighting up. Imagine that when you decide to finish the experiment, you reach out and find there are no cigarettes available. Immediately you will panic and start fumbling around in pockets and drawers, handbags and the like in a frenzied search for nicotine. It's an uncomfortable feeling and one we smokers soon learn to avoid.

That panic feeling smokers get when they are out late at night and supplies are running low starts before they actually run out and gets worse when they are actually smoking the last one. You do a mental calculation: 'I'm going to be at this party for at least two hours, but I've only got four cigarettes.'

You ration your supply as if it were as precious as water and you were crossing the Sahara. You sense the party is coming to an end. It's ending mainly because from the moment your panic started, you have done nothing but remind everyone that you must leave by such and such a time. The party was prevented from being a complete and utter bore from the outset, because you met this fascinating man. He just happened to be the only other smoker there.

Initially it didn't bother you that he was one of those smokers who could take cigarettes or leave them. And you could overlook the fact that he hadn't considered it necessary to bring any cigarettes of his own. His fascination began to wear thin when he began to lecture you about the level of your consumption, particularly as he was matching yours and smoking your cigarettes, which was the only reason you were running low. However, by far his most annoying attribute was that without actually specifically saying so, he managed to imply that he was only smoking so much because of your bad example!

Of course you were far too polite to point any of this out. Once you'd discovered how low you were, there were going to be no more hand-outs. Eventually this boring man took the hint and evaporated. You now feel it's safe to extract your second to last cigarette. As you do, he reappears like a bolt from the blue and without waiting for your reply starts to reach for that precious last cigarette with:

'Do you mind if I have one?'

'Mind! Miiind! You ignorant, stupid idiot! Of course I mind!'

But that's only what you are thinking. He's hit a raw nerve, and you don't want to lose face. What you actually say is: 'Of course I don't mind. I'm like you, I can take them or leave them.' Your sarcasm goes over his head and your last cigarette goes into his mouth. You are left stranded.

So let's be clear: smokers suffer no physical pain whatsoever when they try to 'give up', and provided they want to stop, the 'habit' is easy to break.

This applies not just to you but to all smokers. However, it is an undeniable fact that the vast majority of smokers find it exceedingly difficult, if not impossible, to stop. The reason is fear, panic, and that uncomfortable feeling of wanting a cigarette and not being allowed to satisfy the craving. And let's not blind ourselves to the fact that the panic is real. Smokers will willingly give a cigarette or even their last Rolo to a complete stranger, but if that stranger asked for their last cigarette, the reply, if there is no fear of losing face, would more likely be: 'You are welcome to a pint of my blood. I might even donate one of my kidneys, if you ask me nicely, but my last cigarette? No way!!!'

The only torture smokers suffer either before or after they decide to 'give up' is wanting a cigarette but not being allowed to smoke one. In other words, not being allowed to satisfy the 'craving'. That torture is purely mental, but it's still real and how do you know when or if it will ever end? Mental it might be, but that still makes it exceedingly difficult to 'give up'! NO IT DOESN'T!

Let's take a closer look at the 'willpower' method. It starts with a feeling of doom and gloom with our hoping that, provided we have sufficient willpower, we can endure the misery long enough to be free. But why should we be miserable? After all, we decided that we no longer wanted to smoke. Why aren't we over the moon because we don't have to? Perhaps you feel it's because of that panic feeling we've been discussing. But that doesn't explain it. We've already established that smokers only get that panic feeling when they want to smoke but aren't allowed to. So why should you get it when you've decided that you never want to smoke again?

Perhaps you believe it is because nicotine is an addictive drug, and that the addict has no choice but to continue to crave the drug for an indefinite period after abstention. This sounds very logical, but doesn't in fact explain anything.

What does 'craving' mean? In this context it means nothing more or less than: 'I want a cigarette!' But I've just decided that I never, ever want another, so why am I still craving one? In fact it's completely illogical. Imagine the following conversation between two friends over a coffee:

A: 'I'd love to come shopping with you on a Saturday.'

B: 'I'd really love you to join me. I hate shopping alone.'

A: 'But I have to watch John play soccer. It's so boring. He's too old anyway and I just stand there in the wind and rain terrified that he'll break his leg. And that's the best part! The worst is having to listen to those childish songs after the match.'

B: 'Well it's high time he grew up, and you're just as bad for encouraging him.'

A: 'You're absolutely right, of course. I keep threatening to let him get on with it alone. I've made up my mind – I'm coming shopping with you!'

Now try to imagine A the following Saturday, miserably dragging herself from shop to shop, saying:

'Sorry B, but I've got this terrible urge to rush over to the game. I'm desperately trying not to give in to it. I hope I don't have to go through this torture every Saturday.'

I have a vivid imagination, but in my wildest dreams I wouldn't respond like that, even though personally I hate shopping and love watching sport. You might feel that the example I've given bears no relation to a 'willpower' attempt to 'give up' smoking. But you must have heard smokers say: 'That's it! I'm completely sick of this filthy habit. I'm spending a fortune just for the privilege of destroying myself. I'm "giving up"!' Why else would 'giving up' smoking be the most common New Year's resolution? And don't they then go ahead and spend the next few hours, days and weeks saying: 'I could murder for a cigarette!'?

You've possibly been through this completely illogical process yourself. I did on numerous occasions. 'Addiction' is just a word we use to describe it. But using that word does no more to explain why otherwise intelligent people act so stupidly than saying: it's a habit!

So why do we act so irrationally? The key lies in the expression 'giving up'. When A had the tricky problem of explaining to John that he was about to lose her support, I very much doubt she would have said 'I'm "giving up" coming to watch you.'

You might have noticed that I always put inverted commas round 'give up', and that I only use this expression when I'm referring to a 'willpower' method. Smokers might dislike being smokers and think it illogical that breathing filthy and lethal fumes into their lungs can be pleasurable, or can help them to concentrate, or can relieve boredom or stress, but the fact is that all of them believe that they get some pleasure or a crutch from smoking.

The very expression 'give up' implies sacrifice. You don't have to understand the reason why some foods taste better than others, or why your thumb hurts when accidentally you hit it with a hammer, or why a bulb lights up when you press the light switch. In just the same way you don't have to know why cigarettes appear to improve meals and other social occasions or how they help you to concentrate and to relieve boredom and stress – all you know is that they do.

It seems indisputable that when smokers light up, they feel more relaxed and less distressed than they did the moment before.

If you believe this to be so before you put out what you hope will be your final cigarette, why should you stop believing it after you've finished it? Is it any surprise that after that cigarette, when the phone rings or the tension is high, your brain urges you to light up? And when your friends light up after a meal and you are not allowed to, aren't you going to feel that it is you who is missing out? Of course you hope that time will solve the problem. But why should it? Doesn't absence just make the heart grow fonder? With the 'willpower' method you hope that one day you will wake up shouting EUREKA! I'VE KICKED IT! I'M FREE!

But it rarely ever happens. I'm not saying that a minority don't succeed. Some of them will even enthuse about being non-smokers and will tell you genuinely that they don't miss smoking in the slightest. It is time that solves their problem. All that happens is that if they can abstain for long enough, they gradually accept the situation and the cravings become so few and far between that being a non-smoker becomes acceptable. However, of the minority who succeed in 'giving up', the majority will confess that they do miss the special cigarette, like the one after a meal.

It is these complaining stoppers who make the rest of us frightened to try stopping, by creating this myth of once a smoker always a smoker and that you can never be completely free. Incidentally, have you noticed how these self-righteous ex-smokers are far more vociferous than non-smokers if they get a whiff of your tobacco in a restaurant? It's not really that they object so much, but more a self-protective measure. That whiff reminds them that they are no longer allowed to smoke, and humiliating you helps to reinforce their decision to stop.

'Willpower' methods are so difficult for most smokers and impossible for others because we've been brainwashed from birth to believe that they are so difficult. And if you do pluck up enough courage to try one of these methods, the attempt, far from exploding the belief, simply confirms it to be true. This, incidentally, is why smokers will only make a serious attempt to stop about once every five years. It takes that long for the memory of the misery of the attempt to fade.

When you do succeed with Easyway, you will naturally want to help your smoking friends benefit from it. Don't become frustrated if they don't seem too enthused by your good news. This reluctance might be due to scepticism, or the belief that Easyway might have worked for you but won't for them. Even if they believe you, if they have recently failed a 'willpower' attempt, to ask them to try Easyway would be like trying to persuade a marathon runner who has collapsed a hundred yards short of the finish line to take half an hour's rest and then start all over again.

However, the main difficulty with the 'willpower' method is the sheer doubt and uncertainty. We start off hoping, rather than believing or knowing, that we will succeed. This is negative thinking. Learning to swim can be a difficult and frightening process, but have you ever witnessed the euphoria of a child who has just learned? It might only have been a couple of yards, ending in the child spluttering and swallowing half the pool. But that doesn't diminish the euphoria. That child knows with absolute certainty that it remained afloat under its own steam, without assistance. It can swim! It also knows that, with practice, it will complete a full width, and there'll be more excitement when it does. Only an Olympic gold medal will compare with the euphoria of those first few strokes and the certainty that the child won't go through life never being able to swim.

If your objective is to go a whole year without smoking, it is blatantly obvious that you cannot possibly succeed before the year is up. If your objective is to go your whole life without a cigarette, it is equally obvious that you cannot possibly succeed before your life is up. Which means: even if you do succeed, you won't live to know it! Not much of a prospect, is it, going through life hoping not to fail and knowing that you will never know success. And, of course, the other great drawback of the 'willpower' method is that the smokers using it believe they are making a genuine sacrifice. True, they are in no doubt that the disadvantages of being a smoker far outweigh any advantages. Nevertheless they do genuinely believe that they get some pleasure and/or crutch from smoking. All it takes is just one careless or drunken moment, and they find themselves back in the trap. Little wonder it is so difficult to stop when using 'willpower' methods.

In the previous chapter I asked you to give some thought to the question: 'How do you know when you have succeeded?' I then went into great detail exploding the suggestions made by our clients. You might have noticed that I failed to come up with any brilliant offering myself. Indeed, I have just implied that it is impossible for anyone to be certain that they will never smoke until their life has ended. So how could Debbie, or even Allen Carr himself, know they will never smoke again?

If you asked a trapper, 'Can you state categorically that you will never get your foot caught in a bear trap?' the answer would probably be 'no'. But change the question slightly: 'Could you state categorically that you will never DELIBERATELY get your foot caught in a bear trap?'

The politest reply you would be likely to get is: 'What sort of half-wit would deliberately step on a bear trap?' A trapper might go through life in fear of accidentally stepping on a bear trap, but no way does he worry about deliberately doing so, particularly if he once fell into the trap!

Perhaps you find this comparison of the bear trap and smoking weak. It is if you compare it with smokers who are trying to stop using a 'willpower' method. After all, they genuinely believe that they are 'giving up' a genuine pleasure and/or crutch. And if they are miserable and suspect that the misery is permanent, they might well choose to smoke again. In fact over 90 percent of them do. But imagine you had got hooked on the latest legal drug craze and had been lucky enough to stop. Do you think you would worry about getting hooked again? No doubt you have already heard about this drug craze. It's called:

DEVASTATION

6 Devastation

'Devastation' is an extract from a plant that is indigenous to South America and belongs to the same genus as deadly nightshade. It is one of the most addictive drugs known to mankind. Just one dose will get you hooked. Over 60 percent of the adult natives of the tribes who use this drug become hooked. It is a powerful poison and is used commercially as an insecticide. It gradually breaks down the immune system, causes breathlessness and lethargy and kills one in three of its victims. It tastes bad and systematically destroys the nervous system, causing a feeling of insecurity and lack of confidence. It costs the addict an average £100,000/$131,000 over a lifetime. What does it do for them? Absolutely nothing. What high or buzz do they get from it? Absolutely none.

If you knew and believed the facts about 'Devastation', could I persuade you to try it? Even the most adventurous, fearless or stupid of us wouldn't take just one experimental dose if we believed it would addict us. But supposing you were brainwashed and conditioned from birth into believing that the drug had distinct advantages, and that the downside only took effect if you became hooked and that, far from one dose hooking you, it took years to become hooked? In these circumstances the adventurous among us might try it. Now suppose you were hooked for years and could see the drug clearly as I have described it and you were totally fed up with it. Supposing, too, that you were lucky enough to discover a method that would release you immediately, easily and permanently. Would you hesitate to use that method? And if you found out that it worked,

WOULD YOU DELIBERATELY STEP INTO THE TRAP AGAIN?

I've no doubt that by now you have surmised that the drug I described is our old friend and crutch nicotine. You might well challenge some of the facts I presented. In particular, that it 'systematically destroys the nervous system, causing a feeling of insecurity and lack of confidence' and that it does 'absolutely nothing' for you. However, for the moment, please just accept my description as fact. Read it again, this time trying not to relate it to smoking. Now, do you believe for one second you'd continue to crave cigarettes if the following were true of you?:

- You could perceive smoking purely as the drug I have described.

- You knew that smoking did the opposite of relaxing you, helping your concentration, giving you courage and confidence or relieving stress and boredom.

- You knew that in order to escape all you had to do was never to light another cigarette.

- That whenever the subject of smoking entered your head, you thought 'Eureka! I've kicked it! I'm free!' and not 'I'd love a cigarette' or 'When will I be free?'.

The craving for the cigarette is like a poisoned chalice to the smoker, a mixture of nectar and poison. Smokers want and/or need the nectar, but can't get it without drinking the poison. If any smoker were to list all the advantages and disadvantages of being a smoker and allocate points out of ten to each item, the total point count of the disadvantages would far outweigh the advantages. So why, when our rational side tells us we shouldn't smoke, do we continue to do it? It is because there is a third ingredient in the bottle: Addiction – a mystical force that over-rules our rational side.

A good conjuror can mystify us and make his tricks seem like magic. But once a trick is explained, the mystique disappears. The beautiful truth is that there is no nectar in the bottle.

Easyway explains the mystery of addiction and how it fools its victims into believing they get some form of genuine pleasure or crutch from smoking. When you see smoking without the brainwashed perception, as it really is, as you would see heroin or even 'Devastation', and when you know there is absolutely nothing to give up, only marvellous benefits to receive, you won't have a feeling of doom or gloom or sacrifice. By the end of the book, you'll be impatient to go through the ritual of the final cigarette and, after it, knowing that you are already a non-smoker and enjoying being one.

Smoking is the most subtle, ingenious trap that mankind and nature have combined to lay. Many smokers believe they smoke because they choose to. It is true that no one can force us to smoke. Nevertheless, it is equally true that we don't choose to become smokers. Once you understand the trap completely, you will automatically be free and will no more desire to smoke again than a trapper would deliberately step on a bear trap.

So, why don't I just explain the mystique of addiction and get on with it? Because at this stage you wouldn't believe me. How can I convince you that there's not a smoker in history who has received some genuine crutch or pleasure from smoking? To explain the illusion is simplicity itself, but you will not believe the explanation unless I can first prove the falsity of the 'established' facts about smoking which from birth we have been brainwashed to believe. However, there is a more pressing matter that we must address first. If it can work for any smoker,

WHY DOESN'T EASYWAY WORK FOR EVERY SMOKER?

7 *Why Doesn't Easyway Work For Every Smoker?*

Imagine yourself as a teenager wandering through the gates of a large public garden and finding it so nice that you don't want to leave. As the years pass you begin to suspect that the fruit in the garden, which has been providing you with sustenance, has also been poisoning you. You are not unduly concerned, even though the cumulative effects of the poisoning are apparent in many of the other people who live in the garden with you. You are reassured because these people appear to be reasonably intelligent, just like you. Occasionally, some people do leave, but the vast majority of them choose to return sooner or later.

Eventually you reach the stage where you too would like to leave. You discover that the garden is a giant maze and that the only exit is also the only entrance. There are twenty junctions in the maze. In order to escape you need to guess the correct direction at each one of these junctions. The odds against you getting this right are slightly over a million to one. You try, make just one mistake and remain in the maze. You try again. The problem is you don't know where you made your mistake. You just wander around getting nowhere, not knowing how many decisions you are getting right or wrong. Eventually you decide there is no point even trying.

Does the analogy remind you of a smoker using a 'willpower' method to stop? It is in fact very similar.

Now just suppose there was an official plan of the maze that was said to show the correct way at each junction. You would probably think, 'If I had this plan, escaping from the maze would be a simple matter.' But what if this plan, although written by established and respected experts, gave the wrong information at each junction? You would find it extremely difficult, if not impossible, to escape.

This is virtually the situation confronting smokers when they attempt to escape from the nicotine trap. Smokers, together with the established 'experts' who advise them, believe they know all there is to know about smoking. Let's spend some time testing the knowledge they have imparted to you.

I would like you to respond to the following questionnaire as you believe the majority of people would respond to it, and answer 'yes' or 'no' as appropriate. Don't worry about what you personally believe; put that aside. For the next few minutes you are representing the silent majority.

Personally I hate answering questionnaires, so don't think I'm expecting you to conduct market research or over-tax your brain. Also I won't be marking your answers. That's not the point of this exercise. Just give it your best shot:

QUESTIONNAIRE

1. Do smokers smoke because they choose to?

2. Do people smoke out of habit?

3. Are long-term smokers more hooked than teenagers?

4. Are heavy smokers more hooked than casual smokers?

5. Do youngsters start smoking to feel adult, cool or rebellious?

6. Are smokers stupid?

7. Do smokers enjoy the taste of some cigarettes?

8. Do some cigarettes – e.g. after a meal – taste better than others?

9. Does smoking help to relieve boredom?

10. Does smoking help you to concentrate?

11. Does smoking help you to relax?

12. Does smoking help to relieve stress?

13. Do smokers enjoy smoking?

14. Do some people have addictive personalities?

15. Does smoking help to reduce weight?

16. Does it help to use nicotine gum, patches or sprays?

17. Does it take willpower to stop?

18. Is it necessary to suffer from physical withdrawal symptoms?

19. Do ex-smokers have to endure an initial period of craving and irritability?

20. Is it difficult to stop?

No doubt your answers are a mixture of Yes's and No's. Astonishingly 'No' is the correct answer to all of these questions. Now to the main point of the exercise. I put a similar questionnaire to a representative number of the world's leading 'experts' at the Tenth World Conference on Tobacco or Health held in 1998 in Beijing. On average they got over 75 percent of the answers wrong.

Each piece of advice that these 'experts' give smokers to help them 'give up' is equivalent to the official plan of the maze. It is easy to see why most smokers find it difficult, if not impossible, to give up when you realize that the advice they are getting, and relying on, is wrong.

I claim that Easyway will enable 100 percent of smokers to stop easily, immediately and permanently. So why don't 100 percent succeed? Because it is not easy for all smokers to understand and/ or to follow all the instructions. In the maze analogy, even if you take only one wrong turn you will remain in the maze. When it comes to smoking, to ignore one or more of the instructions will not necessarily prevent you from quitting or even from finding it easy to stop. But it will make it less easy and enjoyable and render you more likely to fall into the trap again.

It is correct to say that with Easyway you cannot fail if you follow all of the instructions. I occasionally receive letters that say something like:

'I understood and agreed with everything you said and followed all your instructions. I even bought some patches, but I'm still smoking.'

Needless to say, one of the instructions is not to use any substitutes, particularly anything containing nicotine. Possibly you are now worrying that there will be dozens of complicated instructions and that you have to be an Einstein to understand them all. Not so; there are only a few instructions to follow while you read the book. The first and most challenging is to:

KEEP AN OPEN MIND

Possibly you are now sitting there with a smug look on your face, thinking: 'If that's the most difficult instruction, this is going to be a doddle!' If so, beware – you are probably already doomed to fail. Try asking your friends if they are broad-minded. See if you can find just one of them to say something like: 'Not in the least, on the contrary, I'm rather narrow-minded.' You must have noticed how incredibly biased and prejudiced everybody else in the world is. Isn't it incredible that it's only you and I who are completely open-minded, never jump to conclusions, and wouldn't dream of making a judgement without knowing all the facts and hearing both sides of the story? Don't underestimate the brainwashing. It is powerful. You not only need to be sceptical about what I tell you, but must question your own views and the facts that you've been brainwashed by the 'experts' to believe.

The second instruction – and second most difficult – is to:

MAINTAIN A HAPPY FRAME OF MIND THROUGHOUT

I'm aware that your smoking problem might well have reduced you to a very bad frame of mind and that you might be terrified of failure. So how can I expect you to be optimistic at this stage? Let me remind you that you are in the enviable position of having a great deal to gain and absolutely nothing to lose. The worst that can happen is that you don't succeed, in which case you will have lost nothing.

Some people believe that Easyway is just an exercise in positive thinking. You know the sort of thing: tell yourself that you can do it and you will. It is more than that. I have always been a positive thinker, purely because it seems logical to be one. It's pretty obvious that you are not likely to achieve anything if your attitude at the outset is, 'I can't do it'. But you are not guaranteed success either if your attitude is, 'I can and will'. In other words, in spite of our attempts to think positively we fail to 'give up' smoking because we are still using 'willpower' methods.

If you doubt this, ask yourself if you have to use a positive outlook not to inject yourself with heroin, or snort cocaine or pop an amphetamine. Is it more realistic to say you simply don't want these things and never will?

Easyway is guaranteed to work for anyone who follows all the instructions, and the more your smoking has dragged you down, the more likely you are to do this. So, put all negative thoughts aside. Regard Easyway as an exciting challenge: to achieve what every smoker on the planet secretly longs for:

TO ESCAPE FROM NICOTINE SLAVERY

The third instruction is:

DON'T ATTEMPT TO STOP OR CUT DOWN BEFORE FINISHING THE BOOK

This point has already been briefly addressed in Chapter 2. The reasons for this instruction will become apparent in due course.

Your fourth instruction is:

DON'T JUMP THE GUN

By this I mean that you must read the book in the sequence in which it has been written – under no circumstances should you jump ahead. By all means go back to previous passages in order to re-read, refresh your memory or to clear up any doubts. In particular, you will find it helpful occasionally to re-read the above instructions and with each one ask yourself, 'Am I really following this instruction or just going through the motions?'

These instructions are easily accessible at any time and you'll find them listed at the back of the book. Just in case you think I've forgotten one, I'll deal with number five in a moment. Before I do, I'd like to remind you of the title of this chapter:

WHY DOESN'T EASYWAY WORK
FOR EVERY SMOKER?

The answer is simplicity itself: follow the instructions. There are only five of them and they are not that difficult or complicated. All you have to do to obtain the feeling of euphoria that Debbie did is to follow them. Debbie was very generous in giving all the credit to me and very modest in ignoring her own contribution. I don't make it easy to stop smoking. The beautiful truth is that it is easy to stop smoking. This is fact. All I do is give you a set of instructions to explain how you too can find it easy to stop. All you need do is follow the instructions.

Now, you might well be thinking:

'Let's not get carried away, Debbie was only into her second week when she wrote that letter. Who's to say she's not puffing away again right now?'

You are absolutely correct. I don't mean Debbie is puffing away, but you are correct in thinking that she might be. There can be two distinct phases of failure. The first is not to achieve the euphoria. The second is to achieve it and still get hooked again.

Undoubtedly one of the most intelligent and certainly the nicest person to attend my centre in the early days was Emma Freud. She kindly volunteered to do the introduction to my video. Her words are worth repeating:

'The only thing in my life I've ever really regretted was the day aged fourteen when I smoked my first cigarette. Twelve years later, I was smoking twenty a day and loved it, actually relished it, but was terrified about what it was doing to my health. Every time I opened the paper I would find an article about cancer or the effects of smoking. I'd turn the page as quickly as I could. Every time somebody told me I was killing myself on tobacco, I'd light another cigarette. I loved it, but I hated it; and the thing that made it even worse was when a friend of mine went to a therapist and gave up completely and effortlessly, overnight.

'We started smoking together. She smoked just as much as me, enjoyed it just as much as me, and yet she could give up and I couldn't. A couple of weeks after she did it, three more of my friends went to see the same therapist and with no great announcement or blowing of trumpets, quietly gave up. They didn't put on any weight. They had no withdrawal symptoms. They didn't lecture me. They had left the club and I hadn't. By the time seven of my friends had given up easily and completely with this man, I couldn't ignore him anymore.

'The time I spent with Allen Carr on December 10th 1988 was some of the most important and effective since that first cigarette when I was fourteen. A lot of people have asked me since what he says that can make you stop so easily. All I can say is: it would take hours to explain, and give them his phone number. If it didn't sound so embarrassing I'd tell you that it changed my life. He is extraordinary. It's really easy and it really, really works and you don't put on any weight. Have fun!'

I'm sure you can forgive me for believing that she was one smoker I thought would never get hooked again. But she did.

This subject has to be addressed, but not here. I like to face things in the correct sequence. Since you cannot lose the euphoria, unless and until you have achieved it, let's first concentrate on how to become a happy non-smoker. In the final chapter we'll discuss how to remain one for the rest of your life.

However, this is an opportune moment to deal with your fifth instruction. It is to:

RECORD YOUR 'PERSONAL STATEMENT'

What is your 'Personal Statement'? Every smoker – man or woman – is confined in exactly the same prison. The key to release from this prison is to remove the brainwashing. The object of Easyway is to remove the brainwashing of every smoker. But just as there are actual differences, and distorted differences, between men and women, so each smoker has to contend with his or her individual brainwashing.

I would like you to pause for a moment, and to record your own feelings about smoking: what you think it does for you, why you smoke and why you want to stop. As you read the book and we gradually remove the brainwashing, add to your 'Personal Statement' any points that really hit home to you, and record the page number on which these appear. You might not see the relevance now, but it will help you not to make the same mistake as Emma.

The nicotine trap is the most insidious, ingenious confidence trick that mother-nature and mankind have combined to lay. A good conjuror will never reveal the key to his trick. Why? Because if he does the trick loses its mystique, the illusion is lost and you are left wondering how you were fooled by it in the first place. It's exactly the same with the nicotine trap. Once it's been explained, it is incredibly simple to comprehend. And, like any other confidence trick, once you realize it's a confidence trick, you will never fall for it again. In other words, you will lose your desire to smoke permanently.

If it is that simple, why don't I just explain the nature of the trap? Well, I am, by opening your eyes to the reality. The key is in the questionnaire. Before I made my discovery, no one understood the true nature of the trap. The simplicity of the subject matter has been confused out of all proportion and now appears to be incredibly complicated. The mass of society, including the so-called 'experts', perpetuates these illusions and misconceptions, mostly inadvertently. We believe them. Some of the so-called experts are wolves in sheep's clothing and wantonly, coldly and calculatingly ensure that the current plan to the maze is kept factually incorrect. Before I can ask you to believe the true and simple explanation of the nicotine trap, I need first to convince you that the facts we have been brainwashed with since birth cannot be true.

In other words, my assertion that the correct answer to each question of the questionnaire is 'no' would mean that smokers get no genuine pleasure or support from smoking. It would also mean that it would not be difficult for any smoker to stop. All smokers are aware that there are considerable disadvantages to smoking in terms of loss of health, wealth and energy. So, if I could show you categorically that, not only does smoking provide no pleasure or support whatsoever, but that it is a major cause of stress and boredom and actually impedes relaxation and concentration, I think you will agree that quitting smoking would not only be easy but enjoyable. In fact, it would be no more or less than the drug I described in Chapter 6: Devastation.

Let's take another step down the road to freedom. Let's take a closer look at:

THE BRAINWASHING

8 *The Brainwashing*

At this stage I am not trying to prove that the facts society accepts are definitely wrong. All I want is you to open your mind and ask yourself whether these 'facts' are definitely right. We have already questioned the first myth: that people smoke out of habit. This fact is standing on its head. Smoking only becomes a habit because people smoke and not the other way around.

No one forces smokers to stop, so when a smoker does stop we naturally assume they have done so because they chose to. Most smokers can remember the occasion of their first experimental cigarette. I certainly can. Ironically, the reason we remember is because it tasted bad and made us cough and feel sick. Pleasure did not come into it. And this is what actually springs the trap. Youngsters suffer the illusion that smokers are enjoying themselves, obscuring their natural reaction, which would be: 'How could anyone get hooked on these filthy things?' Little do they realize that by believing in the illusion, they are being hooked just as surely as a fish nibbling at bait.

You could argue that smoking is an acquired pleasure. But hy do we bother to acquire it? Even if you are several years down the line, if you change your brand or have to sponge a freebie, you still have to acquire the taste. And if you've swapped to an extra light brand, you've probably found yourself taping up the tiny holes to get your customary fix. It is indisputable that no one needs to smoke before they fall into the trap. It's only smokers who can't relax, concentrate, enjoy a meal or answer the phone without a cigarette. Next time you are out, take a look at the non-smokers. Are they behaving as they are because they are not smoking?

You might well remember the day you smoked that first 'experimental' cigarette. It was meant to be experimental, but it turned into something much more. Can you remember when you consciously chose to become a permanent smoker, when you decided to smoke every day and would become anxious/uptight/ fidgety if you didn't have cigarettes on you? No smoker does remember. Isn't the reason obvious? We no more chose to become smokers than we chose to speak our native tongue. Smoking is just part of the culture we are brought up in. Eventually most of us dabble and at one time 80 percent of us got hooked.

The truth is that we neither choose to become smokers, nor do we choose to continue to smoke. If we had a choice, why would we find it so difficult to stop? Why would you need to read this book? On the many occasions that I chose to stop, I wasn't able to. Clearly then, we aren't smoking out of choice, but because we aren't able to exercise our choice. Isn't the true position that we are caught in a trap from which we don't know how to escape? True, there are no iron bars and there's no jailer – other than ourselves – to prevent our escape. Isn't this addiction: when you wish you were free but don't have the power to exercise your choice? Once I discovered the power, I enjoyed exercising my choice immediately and permanently, and so will you.

Because we believe we smoke out of habit, it is logical to assume that the longer you've been a smoker and the heavier you smoke, the more deeply the habit is ingrained. But, again, look at the indisputable facts: it's the longer term, heavier smokers who are stopping, not the younger, casual smokers. Society has failed dismally to prevent its youth from becoming hooked. This applies particularly to young girls. You might argue that young, casual smokers have no need or desire to stop. I can only agree. However, if they are smoking because they are caught in a trap and not because they choose to, who is more effectively hooked? Is it the person who believes they smoke out of choice, or the person who believes they are trapped? Unless you realize that you are in a trap, you'll have no desire to escape from it, and if you have no desire to stop, your chances of stopping smoking are zero. Acknowledging that you are in a trap doesn't guarantee your escape, of course, but it keeps the possibility alive.

Ask yourself, or any smoker, why they smoke and you'll get statements like:

'I enjoy the taste, particularly the one after a meal.'

Do you, or they, actually eat or even chew the cigarette? How does taste actually come into it? And even if it does, how can an identical cigarette out of the same packet taste different on certain occasions? I know you'll be at a loss for an answer. You don't label each cigarette in a packet as 'breakfast', 'with my coffee' or 'after a meal'. Smokers will tell you that a cigarette helps to relieve boredom and stress, and assists concentration and relaxation. But, wait, boredom and concentration are opposites, as are stress and relaxation. Now these smokers aren't stupid and neither are you. If I tried to sell you a magic pill that had the opposite effect to an identical pill taken an hour earlier, you would regard me as either a quack or a really dumb person. Yet society in general, and smokers in particular, seem quite happy to accept that tobacco confers these contradictory 'benefits'.

So why do we accept these contradictions? Why would we be contemptuous of the person attempting to sell us the magic pill, yet be so naive as to accept, believe and actually make those claims about the contradictory benefits of smoking? And why do we do so even when we are fully aware that our little friend or support is incredibly expensive and has awful side effects?

And the contradiction goes even further. You won't find a parent in Western society who doesn't discourage their children from smoking, and parents who are also smokers will do so more vehemently than parents who have never smoked. Yet those same parents will spend hours telling you – usually within earshot of their children – about the pleasure or support they get from smoking.

Why the apparent hypocrisy? It's not really hypocrisy; all smokers sense that they smoke because they have fallen into a trap, not because they choose to.

One of the reasons that I want you to continue to smoke at this stage is because you can't check out the truth about smoking once you've stopped. At the moment, because you believe you get some marvellous pleasure from smoking, if you still believe that when you stop, then you'll go on believing it for the rest of your life. Once you know you get no pleasure from it, then you know you won't be missing it for the rest of your life. If deep down you believe that cigarettes taste marvellous and that smoking is enjoyable, check it out for yourself. Light one up now. Concentrate on taking six deep inhalations and ask yourself what it is that you are actually enjoying. The key here is to concentrate on every single aspect of the cigarette in your hand as it goes to your mouth and you breathe in the smoke.

It's more difficult to do this exercise than we could possibly have imagined. This is because we smoke the vast majority of cigarettes automatically. Even the illusion of enjoyment would disappear if every time you smoked you were consciously aware of breathing unhealthy fumes into your lungs, that this might just be the one cigarette to trigger cancer in you, and that you were going to spend a small fortune in your lifetime on cigarettes.

This, of course, explains the hypocrisy, the double standards and why otherwise honest people have to lie to themselves and others about smoking. It's not deliberate deceitfulness, rather a question of having no choice. It's about holding a busy life together with the apparent aid of cigarettes and seeking to justify motives for smoking by using well-established reasons.

The many reasons we rely upon have been used again and again and, in the case of women, are virtually tried and tested for them by other women smokers. Women generally are so successful at networking, sharing ideas and giving advice from a very early age that the success of the excuses is phenomenal. As a woman passes through her life she will use the excuses pertinent to her at a particular stage to continue smoking, and all the while her smoker friends will be there to reinforce the excuses.

When a relationship fails, cigarettes are used as consolation. When the stresses and strains in a committed relationship surface, cigarettes are there apparently to stop a frantic pulling out of hair or to represent time out from the emotional roller-coaster. And in the later years, when the female body is going through the natural changes of life, creating a state of hormonal imbalance, women smokers will swear that cigarettes are absolutely essential to restore that balance. But, at every turn of the wheel of time, these are excuses and excuses they will remain. Excuses that mask the real truth. After all, who wants to stand among their peers and declare that they feel miserable and have come to the conclusion:

I'M A FOOL! STOP DOING IT!

But this raises an even more frightening spectre: the fear of 'giving up' and of life without cigarettes. So we compromise: 'I will give up, but not today. Today would not be a good time to make the attempt.' In the meantime, there is no point in making ourselves miserable by reminding ourselves how stupid we are being every time we light up, so we close our minds to the truth. We like to smoke at times of stress, relaxation, celebration, boredom and concentration. What other times are there? Only when we are eating, which for most smokers is their favourite cigarette, or when we are sleeping and can't smoke anyway. It never seems to occur to us that there will never be a right time to 'give up'. This is one of the ingenuities, not only of the nicotine trap but of all drug addiction: it is designed to keep you trapped for life.

I haven't at this point proved that smokers get no pleasure or support from smoking. But if you have opened your mind, you will agree that the 'facts' society has brainwashed us to believe about smoking just don't add up. These 'facts' amount to confusion, contradiction and cliché. Even a cursory examination reveals this. So what is the truth? Let's take a closer look at:

NICOTINE ADDICTION

9 *Nicotine Addiction*

The tobacco plant is of the same genus as deadly nightshade. It is a powerful poison and is used commercially as an insecticide. When it is handled in laboratories, the scientists are dressed in anti-contamination suits not dissimilar to those used in the handling of nuclear waste. A large bottle of this type of insecticide (15 ml: the size of a bottle of eye drops) has to be licensed. You cannot buy a whole gram of nicotine on the street like you could a gram of heroin.

Currently more than five million people die annually as a result of nicotine addiction. It might surprise you to learn that this figure has been increasing every year. The World Health Organization estimates that by the 2020s, the number of deaths will be in excess of 10 million yearly.

The average packet of twenty cigarettes contains .5 milligrams of nicotine per cigarette. It takes 1000 milligrams to make 1 gram. If you were to inject the nicotine content of just one cigarette directly into a vein, you would die. Please take my word for this and on no account test it out.

Nicotine is by far the most powerful, addictive drug known to mankind. At one time over 80 percent of the adult male population of Western society was addicted to it. Every puff on a cigarette delivers, via the lungs to the brain, a small dose of nicotine that acts more rapidly than a dose of heroin injected directly into a vein. If it takes you twenty puffs to smoke a cigarette, with just one cigarette you take twenty shots of nicotine.

As soon as the cigarette is put out the nicotine starts to leave the body rapidly and the smoker begins to experience withdrawal symptoms. Smokers believe withdrawal symptoms are the terrible trauma they suffer when they try to 'give up'. The actual physical withdrawal symptoms from nicotine are so slight as to be hardly noticeable. It is an empty, insecure feeling, almost identical to a hunger for food. We learn to recognize that feeling of needing to do something with our hands and interpret it as, 'I want or need a cigarette'.

Within thirty minutes of extinguishing a cigarette, levels of nicotine in the bloodstream drop by half, and to a quarter after an hour. This explains why the majority of smokers smoke about twenty cigarettes a day. Immediately after lighting the next cigarette, the nicotine is replaced and the empty, insecure feeling disappears. This creates the pleasant feeling that smokers describe as enjoyable, satisfying or relaxing. It's rather like removing a pair of tight shoes. Youngsters tend to describe it as a 'hit' or a 'buzz'. Why the difference in the description? Because when we are learning to smoke, no way can the experience be described as pleasurable.

I refer to that empty, insecure feeling as the 'little monster'. Why the 'little monster'? Because although a genuine physical aggravation, it is so imperceptible as to be hardly noticeable. The truth is that 99.99 percent of smokers have lived and died without even realizing that the 'little monster' exists. For years I described myself as a nicotine addict. I also described myself as a golf addict. In neither case did I believe that I was addicted to a drug. I thought nicotine was just a brown and somewhat dirty substance that stained my fingers and teeth. Certainly I never suspected that trying to feed the insatiable appetite of the 'little monster' was the only reason that made me and every other smoker light up.

Don't worry if at this stage you are having difficulty accepting this concept.

You're probably thinking, 'Surely if it were this simple Allen Carr wouldn't have been the only one to have worked it out?' But a clever conjuring trick only becomes obvious once the trick is explained. Before Copernicus, when you watched the sun rise in the east and set in the west, it simply reinforced what the 'experts' and everyone else on the planet believed: that the sun moves round the earth. It's obvious; why should you question the fact?

Now we know it was an illusion created by one simply explained misconception. But so powerful was that simple illusion that it took mankind over a million years to explode the myth. Even today, we still visualize the situation as the sun rising in the east and setting in the west rather than the earth spinning on its own axis until the sun comes into or goes out of view.

However, there are several reasons why the nicotine trap is very difficult to see through. The first is that the 'little monster' is just a feeling and, although you can see the effects of a feeling, the feeling itself is invisible. Invisible phenomena, such as electricity, are difficult to understand. The second is that the feeling itself is imperceptible. The third reason is that the feeling is indistinguishable from normal hunger and insecurity, further confusing the situation. The fourth reason, and major cause of the deception, is that it works back to front. It is when we are not smoking that the 'little monster' starts to nag you to light up. And, of course, there is a delay between the last cigarette and the need to light another. But the moment we light up the relief is almost instantaneous. We do feel more relaxed and less distressed than we did a moment before. We don't know how a cigarette performs this little miracle, any more than we know how we get light just by flicking a switch. We don't need to know. All we need to know is that it does. Little wonder that smokers regard a cigarette as a pleasure and a crutch.

Incidentally, this back to front aspect is the key to all drug addiction. Someone who has never been addicted to heroin would be horrified to watch an addict self-inject with the drug. It is blatantly obvious to the onlooker that the addict is not doing this to obtain wonderful hallucinations but to relieve the misery of withdrawal. Another subtle aspect of addiction is that, although it is the first dose that hooks us, the whole process is usually so subtle and gradual that it can take years for us to realize that we are actually hooked. The truth only hits us when we try to stop and find we can't. Even then it doesn't really sink in. Instead we make excuses. 'I picked a bad time' is a favourite. In the beginning we can go days or even weeks and not think about smoking. We would laugh at the thought of getting into a panic if we didn't have cigarettes on us.

Addiction is rather like growing old: it happens so gradually we don't notice it. Each day we feel no different to the way we did the day before, and the face we look at in the mirror every morning is identical to the one we looked at twenty-four hours earlier. However, study a photo of yourself taken ten years ago and change is obvious. It's the same with smoking. We forget that we could enjoy social occasions, concentrate and cope with stress before we got hooked. Even when our lethargic state becomes obvious, we blame it on ageing rather than our little 'friend'.

If only you had a photograph of how well you felt before you fell into the trap! I would love to be able to project you into your mind and body and show you how you will feel only three weeks after extinguishing your final cigarette. And I don't mean just physically or energy-wise. I mean how confident and complete you will feel. You'll be thinking: 'Will I really feel this good?' The only mystery in your life will be why it wasn't obvious to you before. You'll view smokers not with envy but with pity, as you would a heroin addict. Unfortunately, I can't project you forward three weeks – but you can. All you have to do is open your mind, follow the instructions and use your imagination.

Perhaps you have previously 'given up' for three weeks or longer and felt the complete opposite to the state of euphoria that I have just described. If so, I don't doubt you; it happened to me several times. But neither of us was using Easyway.

There is one more ingenious aspect to the nicotine trap that I must address before I can progress to the main topic of this work: women and smoking. This aspect is immunity. Have you ever wondered how wild animals know the difference between food and poison? It's easy for us. If we have sensible parents they'll ensure that we can't get access to poisons until we are old enough to understand what they are. But how do wild animals manage? Mother Nature has equipped all creatures on the planet with various ingenious devices to help them to survive. I know that your cat is a domesticated pet and that you wouldn't dream of feeding her poison. But she doesn't know that. Have you noticed how a cat will first sniff her food when she is not certain about it? She might then sample a minute portion and either tuck in with gusto or eat tentatively. Occasionally she won't touch it and just walk away with her tail in the air as if you had put down poison for her. That's because you had!

Two of the ingenious devices that all creatures possess, including us, are smell and taste. If something smells bad, it's poison. If you are not sure, sample a morsel. If it tastes bad it's poison. The system is so ingenious that even if good food turns putrid, it will smell and taste awful. This is why our first cigarettes and alcoholic drinks taste awful. Our body is telling us: 'You are feeding me poison, please don't!' The lucky ones, for whatever reason, heed the warning and never smoke or drink alcohol again. However, if we persist, Mother Nature doesn't abandon us. She could say: 'Well, I've given you fair warning. If you are too stupid to heed that warning, so be it'. But she doesn't. Instead she gives us a second chance by making us cough and feel increasingly giddy and nauseous, and if we fail to heed that warning she'll ensure that we throw up.

Again, many people believe that a cough, or feeling sick and vomiting are themselves diseases. On the contrary, they are simply symptoms of a disease and are often part of the cure. Coughing and vomiting are two other ingenious survival devices with which Mother Nature has equipped us in order to eject poisons from our lungs and stomachs

Her desire to protect us doesn't end there. If we continue to smoke and drink alcohol on a regular basis, she assumes that we do so because we have no choice, not because we are stupid enough to choose to. Ironically, her assumption is correct. She then triggers yet another survival technique that is a miracle in itself. Let's take a closer look at:

OUR IMMUNE SYSTEM

10 *Our Immune System*

Like most of us I never really gave much thought to my immune system, nor indeed to any aspect of the natural functioning of my body, let alone puberty and growing older, which were never spoken of. I was brought up to believe that the occasional bout of illness was quite normal. But no one expected to contract a permanently crippling or terminal disease prior to reaching old age. On the relatively few occasions that I was ill, I would visit my doctor and he would prescribe a medicine, pill or ointment that would cure me. My immune system got none of the credit.

It wasn't until very late in life that it occurred to me that, provided we hadn't poisoned their habitat, wild animals could survive without doctors. Indeed, the human race had survived for hundreds of thousands of years without the benefit of doctors or their paraphernalia. As any doctor will tell you, by far the most powerful and effective healing force is our immune system: yet another ingenious survival device with which we are equipped.

Our immune system not only fights disease but is so sophisticated that if you continue to poison your body on a regular basis, your immune system will build a partial immunity to the poison. Rasputin was able to survive a dose of arsenic twenty times greater than the dose that would kill an average human being. This was because over time he built an immunity to it. Rats and mice could survive the poison Warfarin after just three generations.

When we teach ourselves to smoke tobacco and drink alcohol regularly, we build an immunity to the bad taste and poisonous effects. In case you are now thinking: 'Great! My immune system will prevent me from contracting lung cancer, emphysema, arteriosclerosis or any of the other killer diseases', bear in mind that you not only build an immunity to the poisonous effects of the drug, which is only partial anyway, but you also build immunity to the drug itself. This requires further explanation.

Just as smokers have good days and bad days, so do non-smokers. In order not to confuse matters, let's assume that before we light that first cigarette we feel OK. Of course, when we smoke that first cigarette we might cough and feel giddy. But again let's ignore the poisonous effects and assume we are still OK. However, when we put out that first cigarette the nicotine will begin to leave our body and we will experience withdrawal. At this stage the empty, insecure feeling is so slight we aren't even aware of it. All we feel is slightly unwell. If we light another cigarette the nicotine will be replaced, the empty, insecure feeling will go and we will feel exactly the same as we did before we lit that first cigarette.

Now this is a mind-blowing concept. And if what I claim is true, it means that the only reason smokers continue to smoke is to feel like they did before they lit the first cigarette. In other words, the only pleasure or crutch anybody ever gets from smoking a cigarette is:

TO FEEL LIKE A NON-SMOKER

The feeling of pleasure or a crutch is real, but it is an illusion to believe that the cigarette should take the credit for it. On the contrary, the cigarette was responsible for the below-par state in the first place. To claim that cigarettes relax you is equivalent to claiming that wearing tight shoes relaxes you. And, of course, that second cigarette doesn't solve the problem. On the contrary, it simply puts more nicotine into your body to cause those withdrawal symptoms that will last for the rest of your life. This is how you can tell the difference between genuine pleasure and drug addiction. I love lobster. But I can go years without eating it and it doesn't bother me in the least if I do. I don't feel insecure or get into a panic when I have no lobster in my presence and I never got to the stage where I didn't feel secure unless twenty lobsters were hanging round my neck! With smoking there is a chain effect. Each cigarette creates the need for the next.

Now back to the immunity. As our body builds immunity to nicotine, we find that we don't quite get back to par when we light up again. We live with a permanent nicotine hangover, a state of discomfort which we believe is normal. Sadder still, we have learned a behaviour which we wholeheartedly believe will get rid of it. Like all other forms of drug addiction, the tendency is to have to light up more often, which simply perpetuates the process. At the same time the poisonous and financial effects are also accumulating. Like all drug addiction the lower it drags you down, the greater your need for what you believe to be your crutch and friend. When I reached the stage of being a chain-smoker, I was completely immune to the effects of the drug and no longer had even the illusion that smoking provided support or pleasure. Physically I was so low that I knew that if I didn't stop I would soon be dead, yet mentally I was so dependent on my 'crutch' that I was prepared to die rather than stop.

This is an apt time to address one of the most important aspects of all addiction. When we are young and fit the health effects don't bother us and, provided we can afford to smoke, we have no particular desire to stop. As we become increasingly immune to relieving the 'little monster', the tendency is to increase the intake and thus exacerbate the problem. A smoker's cough develops and you become increasingly lethargic and breathless. This increases the stress in your life, making you want to smoke more, which in turn increases your health and financial problems. Eventually it dawns on you that you seem to be getting no pleasure from smoking. The initial solution at this stage is to cut down, but you have come to what I refer to as the 'critical point'. It's a stage that all drug addicts eventually reach and it's important that you understand its importance. It's equivalent to the stage that an insect reaches when it is satiated by the nectar in a pitcher plant, wishes to escape, but finds itself stuck and soon realizes the plant was eating him and not vice versa.

At the very time that a part of your brain wants you to smoke more and more, another part wants you to smoke less and less. You are now in the unenviable position of not being allowed to smoke enough and yet smoking too much. From this point on you will not suffer even the illusion of enjoying being a smoker.

If the 'little monster' can reduce a previously happy, healthy youngster to such a state, you might well argue that this monster, far from being little, is of enormous proportions. I refer to him as the 'little monster' because physical withdrawal is not the main problem. As I have already explained, he is so slight that we don't even recognize his existence. We only know him as 'I want a cigarette'.

There are times when you can see the physical effects of withdrawal. Observe smokers who have gone longer than usual without being able to light up. They begin to get restless and fidgety, playing with their lighters or tapping their packet of cigarettes. Eventually their hands will go up to their mouths and they will start to tense their jaw muscles. It's this feeling that smokers describe as needing to do something with their hands. Non-smokers don't have this problem.

I always say to smokers in the early stages of a group session that it's quite obvious they are not quite believing what I am saying. Although we encourage smokers to smoke throughout the session, there usually comes a time when nobody has lit up for a while and no one wants to be the first to do so. They become restless and their hands go up to their mouths. I interrupt what I am saying and point out that they are all now obviously restless. I explain that I am pointing this out not because I am a sadist and want to embarrass them, but for two very good reasons.

First, to make them see the truth: that it's not so much that smokers are relaxed when they are smoking, as that they are decidedly unrelaxed when they aren't.

The second reason is that it is clear to me that not only are they becoming restless, but they are no longer concentrating. This is another reason why I like smokers to continue to smoke until they've finished reading the book. I don't want you sitting there restless and agitated. I want you to be relaxed and absorbing the truths that I am explaining.

Is this an admission that smoking helps you to concentrate? On the contrary, as I will explain later, it is proof that smoking impedes concentration.

Fortunately, you are never badly addicted to the drug itself. The 'little monster' is simply part of the overall illusion, the catalyst that creates the real problem is:

THE 'BIG MONSTER'

11 *The 'Big Monster'*

The 'big monster' is the brainwashing. It is the belief that we get genuine pleasure from smoking or that it provides a crutch; that we will have to exercise massive willpower and go through terrible trauma in order to stop; that if we achieve the impossible and stop, social occasions will never be quite as enjoyable as when we smoked, and we will be less able to handle stress. The 'big monster' is also belief in all those other illusions listed in the questionnaire on page 68. Incidentally, those twenty points are by no means exhaustive.

I now come to what is by far the most difficult part of this book. I have been accused of being arrogant and chauvinistic. The accusations don't bother me too much. I have valid reasons for appearing to be both. My insistence that I am right and all the so-called 'experts' are wrong is born of frustration. Over the years I have witnessed many experts acting in ways that were consistent with the prevailing attitudes to smoking. What shook me was their blinkered attitude to the issue, and their reluctance to embrace a radical and yet obviously effective approach. It is only now, more than twenty years later, that increasing numbers of experts are beginning to realize that it is the psychological state of the individual addict that counts and not the substance itself. My accumulated knowledge of drug addiction comes from more than twenty years of dealing with and answering effectively the questions and worries of the addicted.

The only reason that some smokers don't succeed with Easyway is because they fail to follow all the instructions. The main reason they don't follow the instructions is because they take the advice of a doctor or some other so-called 'expert'.

If I temper my arguments with false modesty, the chances are you will be less likely to believe them and, consequently, less likely to follow all of the instructions.

It would be nice for me to think that the reason I succeeded in cracking the code to the smoking jail was because of my intellect. I know, however, it was a combination of incidents, accidents and deductions that were peculiar to me but would soon be at the disposal of every smoker. It's like the ultimate invention that every household has to have.

I NEVER SUFFERED THE ILLUSION THAT SOME CIGARETTES TASTE GOOD

When I started smoking the 'blends' were less refined and didn't contain sweeteners such as almond oil, vanilla or glycol to moisten your throat to 'help you smoke'. I remember how bad those first cigarettes tasted, yet I quickly became a chain-smoker. No way can a chain-smoker suffer the illusion that the routine of smoking is pleasurable. I've always prided myself on not being a sheep and going my own way. I watched my father coughing and spluttering every morning, and was convinced that he got no pleasure whatsoever from smoking. And I knew that I was a very strong-willed person. In all other areas of my life, I was in control. I wouldn't allow anyone to dominate me. But I was completely dominated by cigarettes, although I loathed them and knew they would soon kill me. Whenever I tried to 'give up', I couldn't concentrate, enjoy life or cope with stress, was completely miserable and yet seemingly powerless to resist the temptation.

Then my son persuaded me to read an extract from one of those family medical books. I couldn't be bothered explaining to him that I already knew that smoking was killing me. I read the extract half-heartedly and found it sheer gobbledegook, with terms such as capillary beds, adrenaline and noradrenaline, biochemical responses, inhibitory cells and the like. But, for some reason that I can't explain, I kept on reading, and went over it again and again. I can only describe the experience as being similar to staring at what appears to be a straightforward image or pattern for a long time and then finding another, separate picture emerging in front of your eyes. Blink your eye and the illusion disappears.

Gradually I began to make sense of the language. The extract informed me that when nicotine leaves the body, smokers suffer an empty, insecure feeling that is only relieved when they light another cigarette.

I blinked not once but several times. Far from disappearing back into the mass of the previous image, the new picture stayed with me and was distinct from that original image. Let me make it clear. I didn't discover that when nicotine leaves the body, smokers suffer an empty, insecure feeling that is relieved when they light another cigarette. Apparently, this process had been known by the medical profession and, incidentally, the tobacco industry, for years and was simply regarded as one of the reasons smokers found it difficult to stop.

My great discovery was to realize that the only reason any smoker continues to smoke is to scratch that 'itch' – not because they enjoy smoking, or because it relaxes them, or improves meals, or relieves stress, or helps them to concentrate. No one would deliberately place their hands in boiling water just to get the relief of removing them. But this is what smokers effectively do. Once they can see this clearly and understand it, they stop immediately and permanently and are happy to do so.

When I started out I believed I could cure any smoker simply by saying: 'Look, the only reason that you smoke is that when nicotine leaves your body, it makes you feel insecure and when you replace it, you feel secure again. In fact, it's like wearing tight shoes just to get the relief of removing them!' How naive of me! It was equivalent to Copernicus saying: 'No, the sun doesn't really move across the sky. The fact is the earth is spinning and this creates the illusion.' And then expecting everyone to take his word for it. The reply he probably got was: 'If the earth was spinning, I'd feel it. The only thing that's spinning is your brain!' The reply I most commonly got was: 'When you tell me you never enjoyed a cigarette, I believe you. Why can't you believe that I do?'

It soon became clear that before I could convince any smoker that what I was claiming was true, I had to remove the brainwashing and the illusions and show them that what they believed wasn't true.

Easyway consists of two parts: one is to remove the brainwashing and the other is to explain the nature of the nicotine trap. Both parts involve communication. It is equally obvious that there are basic differences between the sexes, both physical and emotional.

A combination of two factors prompted this version of the book: one involves good news, the other bad. The bad news is the occasional letters I receive from women whose lives are clearly being ruined by smoking, who obviously desperately want to stop, have made monumental efforts to do so, yet seem unable to succeed.

The good news is the many letters I receive from women like Debbie. They not only inspire and encourage me to continue the battle against nicotine addiction, but I've often thought they would be a tremendous inspiration to those who have so far failed to stop.

I've already stated that Debbie's letter doesn't explain how Easyway works. But what it does show is her frame of mind, and the excitement and exhilaration that will soon be yours too.

That is exactly what we are trying to achieve. Let me remind you that it is not a frame of mind whereby you think: 'I must never, ever smoke another cigarette.' Rather, it is the attitude that someone who has never been addicted to heroin would have towards a heroin addict. When you see a smoker lighting up I want your instant response to be, 'Pity that poor sap! Thank goodness I'm free!', and not 'Pity, I can't just do that occasionally.'

In order to achieve that frame of mind permanently, you need first to remove the brainwashing and see smoking as it really is: nothing more or less than addiction to 'devastation'. We have already removed some of the brainwashing and questioned more. But we need to remove it all. By the way:

WHAT IS YOUR FAVOURITE PERFUME?

12 *What Is Your Favourite Perfume?*

I've always greatly admired women who are fastidious about their appearance. Some women can spend hours – and a small fortune – shopping for the right clothes and accessories, suffer semi-asphyxiation having their hair done, cleanse their teeth and bodies, meticulously apply their make up, ensuring that their perfume is neither cheap nor over-applied. The end result is nothing less than a work of art. But all that effort can be completely ruined by breath that smells like an ashtray. A classic example is actress Joanna Lumley. She is an incredibly beautiful woman who has everything, including the dubious ability to 'light up' and instantly transform herself into 'fag-ash Lil'.

I'm not telling you anything that you don't already know, of course. Let's face it, you may have tried to look the part by standing in front of a mirror and practising how to smoke 'with allure'. There is even a web site devoted to sexy smoking! But when the lens of a camera or camcorder is focused on you, will you pose, pout or try to smoke sexily? Not on your life! Then it's a frantic, 'Where can I stub out my cigarette?'

I receive many letters on this subject: 'I go to all this trouble. I might just as well spread manure all over my body! I can't understand myself. Why am I so stupid?' Don't worry; all women smokers despise themselves, even though many of them cannot bring themselves to admit it, and none of them can understand why they continue to smoke. The reason might appear to be rank stupidity, but really it's fear. It's also another demonstration of the incredible power of nicotine addiction.

Another common theme in the letters I receive from women is the effect that smoking has on their complexion and circulation.

I watched both my father and elder sister suffer painful deaths from cancer caused by cigarette smoking. No doubt many of you have had similar experiences of watching people close to you die from the effects of nicotine, and even after living through their hell, like me you couldn't stop. With lung cancer I thought either you were lucky, and got away with it, or you were unlucky. You probably suspect that I'm now using the doctors' method by trying to frighten you into stopping. Not so; that tactic didn't help me to stop and if it would help you, you would already be free.

But if you knew for certain that the next cigarette would be the one to trigger lung cancer, would you smoke it? If I had been able to see what was actually happening inside my body, I sincerely believe I would have stopped. Now, I'm not referring to my nicotine-stained lungs. The nicotine stains on my teeth and hands didn't bother me unduly, although I know this is another aspect that does bother most women. But it doesn't make them stop! Many will find ingenious ways of masking or hiding the smell of smoke; rubbing slices of lemon onto their fingers in an attempt to get rid of the stains is a favourite.

No, I am referring to the gradual and cumulative gunging up of all your blood vessels. The effect is not unlike that of ingesting one of those modern chemical fertilizers. The fertilizer is actually a poison, but plants that are fed with it in small, measured doses appear to thrive. The reality is that the plant is calling on all its reserves to grow protective layers against the daily doses of the poison. After being given repeated doses the plant gradually starts to show signs of failing, with discoloured leaves, black spots and withering branches. The changes that the poison brings about are all too visible. With smoking the supply of oxygen and nutrients to every organ, muscle and bone in the body is gradually replaced by carbon monoxide and other poisons. I had a permanently grey complexion as a consequence. Sophisticated beings that we are, we don't want to attribute this change to smoking and prefer to explain away our appearance by putting it down to natural colouring or a hectic lifestyle.

Then there's the dried-up look, or you may notice liver spots on your skin, see specks in front of your eyes whenever you stand up quickly, or develop severe varicose veins. All these changes we blithely put down to old age. However, the worst health aspect, I believe, is that the gunging up process also impedes the functioning of the immune system. This is like a bank; it has finite reserves. Keep taking out and you'll discover, to your great cost, that there is no overdraft facility.

We don't need doctors to tell us that smoking causes breath-lessness, asthma, bronchitis, emphysema and other respiratory diseases. We know all this. But our immune system is often overlooked. It's fighting a constant battle against everyday illnesses and diseases, including cancer. If it's defective, it can't do its job properly, and must prioritize. It's like when we take on too much – we can't cope with everything effectively. You observe heavy smokers. You'll find all of them have grey complexions, dry, wrinkled skin and a listless, dull look in the eyes. This is the reality of a lifetime of smoking – if you are LUCKY enough not to have developed a serious illness.

Have you heard those stories about smokers who are warned by their doctors that gangrene will set in and they will have to have their toes amputated if they don't stop? Still they don't stop. They have toes amputated and are then warned that it will be their feet or part of a leg next, unless they stop smoking. Smokers who face this situation know that their doctors aren't bluffing, but still they don't stop! Can you imagine being in that position and still being unable to stop?

No, I don't want to harp on this subject. I promised you that there would be no horror stories and that I have nothing but good news for you. However, it does help to illustrate a very important point. Do you think any smoker would rather have a leg removed than stop because of the wonderful pleasure or crutch they get from smoking?

If you consider Debbie's letter again, why is she so excited and enthusiastic? All that has happened is that she has become an ex-smoker. Have you ever heard a non-smoker enthuse about how her hair and body smells and how great she feels? Make no mistake, Debbie's enthusiasm is genuine. Her great excitement is down to escaping from the genuine misery of being a smoker!

Obviously you will know smokers who have managed to stop without the help of Easyway, and possibly some of them found it relatively easy to do so. Do they enthuse like Debbie and Allen Carr? It's very unlikely. The reason is that they still retain most of the brainwashing. You might have noticed that smokers who wish to stop, or who have succeeded in stopping, always refer to 'giving up'. I do the same when referring to a 'willpower method'. Those smokers truly believe that they have made a genuine sacrifice. Obviously they would rather be ex-smokers than non-smokers, but the majority of them become complaining ex-smokers. You must have heard them: 'I used to love a cigarette after a meal, but I daren't have one now!' With Easyway, I never refer to 'giving up', but to quitting, stopping or, most accurate of all, escaping!

Unfortunately, stories about smokers being prepared to die rather than 'give up' reinforce two of the most stubbornly held beliefs about smoking: that cigarettes are purveyors of great pleasure and/or provide a crutch, and that nicotine addiction exerts an unshakeable hold over its victims. If a smoker threatened with limb amputation still cannot stop, how can Allen Carr expect me to believe that no smoker need suffer from severe nicotine withdrawal symptoms and that any smoker can find it easy to stop? Let's address another subject that seems to affect women more than men:

HUNGER

13 *Hunger*

Why are women generally more concerned with hunger than men? Again, brainwashing is the main cause. For decades women have been targeted with images of the 'ideal' body and 'desired look', and now men are showing signs of falling prey to similar marketing techniques. Body image has become a cultural norm. But more women than men are likely to strive to be that 'ideal' weight or achieve that 'desired' look. Many women use these goals as measures of self-worth, and in many cases how they interact with others is dictated by the degree to which they achieve these goals.

In Western societies food is now designed for our 'convenience'. Supermarkets, powerful food conglomerates and massive advertising campaigns seem to be working together to determine what we eat. Much of the food we devour looks good, fills our bellies and tastes good – and is laden with additives, sugar and salt.

It is 'short-change' food. The manufacturing process it undergoes to look the way it does and to be quick to prepare strips it of the natural energy and nutrients we require. It fails to deliver slow-releasing energy and vitamins to our systems. It robs us of energy. Indeed, our bodies have to work harder trying to find the pathetically small amounts of nutrients contained in them. The phenomenally poor return leaves our bodies in need, and perpetually hungry. Our response to the constant 'I'm hungry' signals is to eat more processed food, which promptly turns to fat.

This is the trap that eating highly refined foods sets for us. Women, because they generally take more pride in their appearance than do men, are usually the ones who try hardest to escape from it. Unfortunately, the methods they choose are often counter-productive. Some women spend much of their lives dieting in order to maintain their figures, trying one fad diet after another. Most of these diets starve the body of the nutrients it needs to keep it healthy. Swapping three modest, nutritious meals for three glasses of some ultra-processed substitute that tastes like embalming clay is not sensible.

We tend to regard hunger as a terrible evil. It isn't. In reality it is just another of Mother Nature's ingenious devices to ensure that we survive whether we like it or not. We have already discussed how wild animals tell the difference between food and poison. But why should wild animals want to eat in the first place? The answer is obvious: because they would die if they didn't. True, but do they know that? Or do they eat because they get hungry?

Let's examine our motives. Obviously we eat because we wouldn't survive if we didn't. But can you remember once in your life saying to yourself: 'It is essential that I eat now, otherwise I will starve to death'? I've no doubt that you have many times said something like, 'I'm dying for something to eat!' or, 'I'm starved. I must eat something!' You don't really mean that you are dying or starving. In reality you are just being over-dramatic. You may at the worst have felt faint or dizzy because of lack of food. What you are really saying is, 'I'm ravishingly hungry and am desperate to satisfy my hunger'. Does a baby cry for food because it knows it will die if it doesn't have it? Obviously not; it cries because it's hungry.

Hunger is a wonderful phenomenon. If you eat meals containing little or no junk food (ie, food in its natural state) at regular times, you won't be hungry until your next meal is due. You then have the pleasure of satisfying your hunger three times a day forever more. Isn't life wonderful? Infinite pleasure with no downside. You might be under the impression that the only food that is good for you tastes like cardboard. Actually the foods that benefit you most taste the best. Hard to believe, but I promise you it's true. (If you remain to be convinced, read *The Easy Way for Women to Lose Weight* or *No More Diets*.)

Even when we are aware of being hungry and, for whatever reason, are unable to satisfy our hunger, what is so bad about that feeling? There's no actual physical pain. Oh, your stomach might be rumbling, but that's not physical pain. In truth it's just an empty, insecure feeling which we only know as: 'I want to eat'. If this feeling is not satisfied, it soon becomes: 'I must eat'. If food is scarce or unobtainable, fear and panic enter the equation and the feeling becomes: 'If I can't obtain food soon, I will die.'

Bear in mind that every natural instinct with which Mother Nature has endowed us is aimed at ensuring our survival. It follows that the fear of death – even when no physical pain is involved – is both real and powerful. This fear is so great that it will force predators to risk injury and death by attacking adult and healthy prey when young or injured prey are not available. We humans will even resort to cannibalism if other types of food are not available to us. Perhaps, like me, you feel that you could not be reduced to that level. But perhaps, also like me, you have never been without food for longer than twenty-four hours at a stretch.

I have said that the craving for nicotine is indistinguishable from a hunger for food. In reality this craving has a more powerful effect. Just as an alcoholic given a handout will buy booze rather than food, so a smoker who cannot afford both will choose tobacco rather than food. This is because on average we have to satisfy our hunger for food only three times a day whereas our craving for nicotine occurs much more frequently. The average twenty-a-day smoker will experience this craving some 7,120 times a year. Understandably, our behaviour is geared to getting rid of the discomfort we experience most often. The nicotine itch takes precedence over anything else.

Some smokers believe they smoke because they enjoy the taste or the ritual. One of the special cigarettes for many smokers is the first of the day. Ironically, it's the one that makes us cough and splutter. In no way can it be described as enjoyable, so why do we smoke it? Because we have gone eight hours without nicotine. We have also gone without food for the same length of time, of course, but the learned response is to satisfy the craving for nicotine first. Although the empty, insecure feeling caused by hunger is indistinguishable from the symptoms of nicotine withdrawal, satisfying one will not satisfy the other.

Imagine the confusion this situation creates in the mind of a smoker. Non-smokers do not have this problem. They also wake up with an empty, insecure feeling, but there is no confusion as to its cause. They know they've gone eight hours without food and are looking forward to breaking their fast. Breakfast is the favourite meal of most non-smokers, simply because the longer you fast the greater the pleasure of relieving it. Having satisfied their hunger and provided their bodies with the energy and nutrients required, they no longer have an empty, insecure feeling and are equipped to enjoy the day.

But smokers wake up with an additional empty, insecure feeling. Twenty-a-day smokers are in the habit of relieving their withdrawal symptoms every hour. For them to be without nicotine for eight hours is equivalent to non-smokers being without food for nearly three days. Little wonder the smoker's first instinct is to light up no matter how bad that experience might be. True, smokers will actually feel less tense than they did a moment before they lit up, but they will have done nothing to relieve the empty, insecure feeling for food. In fact, due to the immunity effect, they will have only partially relieved the craving for nicotine, and the moment they put out that cigarette the nicotine chain starts again. Hence the famous actress's response to the question: 'Do you not think you would feel better if you ate breakfast?' – 'But I do! My breakfast consists of five cigarettes and three cups of coffee!'

If the empty feeling for food and nicotine is identical, how can a smoker ever know what percentage relates to one or the other? And since the craving for nicotine cannot actually be satisfied by smoking a cigarette, it means that a smoker is permanently hungry. Incidentally, this is why the cigarette after a meal is so important to smokers. Non-smokers are completely relaxed once they've satisfied their hunger. It's not so much that a cigarette enhances a meal for smokers, as smokers cannot even enjoy that meal unless and until they can feed the 'little monster'.

Ironically, the situation becomes even more confusing when smokers attempt to stop by using a 'willpower' method. During our smoking lives we've been regularly fooled into lighting a cigarette when what our bodies were really crying out for was sustenance, not poison. In other words we've been in the habit of substituting a cigarette for food. But once we decide to stop, although the nicotine leaves our bodies within a few days, for a period our bodies continue to experience that empty, insecure feeling. We know that feeling as, 'I want or need a cigarette!' This is terribly confusing: we've been listing all the powerful and rational reasons why we should no longer want a cigarette, yet here we are irrationally wanting one. Since we can no longer partially relieve the feeling by smoking, the natural tendency is to reverse the procedure by eating chocolates, sucking boiled sweets or chewing gum. These substitutes won't even partially relieve the 'little monster'. What they will do is coat your teeth with sugar, ruin your appetite, make you put on pounds and leave you feeling miserable and frustrated. The reason? You will sense – without understanding why – that the only thing that will help relieve that empty feeling is a cigarette. You won't allow yourself to have one, though. You will then feel even more deprived and miserable. Your need for the cigarette will intensify, as will your frustration for not being allowed to satisfy that need.

It's a cause and effect situation that can end only one way. Eventually your reserves of willpower are exhausted and you find some excuse to light up without too much loss of face. Once you understand the nicotine trap, the mystery isn't so much why otherwise strong-willed people cannot 'give up' by using willpower, so much as how any smoker manages to succeed using this method.

In fact, only a small percentage of them ever do. Even those who survive the few days necessary without nicotine for the 'little monster' to die are never sure when they are free. Because the empty, insecure feeling is identical to normal hunger and stress, ex-smokers who have 'given up' by using a 'willpower' method will interpret that feeling as, 'I need a cigarette!'. They will do this for weeks, months or even years after their final cigarette and the expiration of the 'little monster'.

If you have followed and understood what I have been saying, you might well be asking yourself how long it takes for the 'little monster' to die, and how will you know when he is dead? I regret that I cannot answer either question. These might appear to be important matters to you, but in fact both are completely irrelevant. An analogy will help you to understand why. Imagine you are involved in a fight to the death under water. You succeed in severing your adversary's oxygen supply. From that moment he is doomed. Does it matter one bit how long it takes him to die or to know the exact moment that he does? Similarly the 'little monster' is doomed the moment you cut off its supply of nicotine. Perhaps you are worrying about suffering during the period that our bodies continue to experience that empty, insecure feeling after cutting off the supply of nicotine. You have no need to. Remember, smokers experience that feeling throughout their smoking lives and it is so slight they don't even realize that it exists. It's only the lack of understanding that causes the confusion and frustration. Once you realize that the empty feeling is caused by the previous cigarette and the one thing that will prevent its relief is another cigarette, that period can be one of exquisite joy rather than misery. However, more about this later (see Chapter 18).

Nowadays smoking is generally regarded as decidedly anti-social. Even smokers themselves seem to concur with this assessment, to the extent that many won't light up in the bedroom and some discipline themselves to eat a little breakfast. Many others won't light up until they leave the house. It always distressed me during my morning jog, particularly in winter, to see young girls dangling a lighted cigarette in their gloved fingers. The brainwashing says they should be happy and sparkling. In reality they look dull, miserable and depressed.

It is its similarity to hunger that makes addiction to nicotine such a powerful force. In both cases you suffer no aggravation whatsoever, until you become aware of either needing food or a cigarette. And, providing you have food that you enjoy and your favourite brand of cigarettes, you can immediately enjoy the pleasure of satisfying your hunger and 'enjoy' relieving the craving. So, in both cases, there appears to be pleasure without any downside.

If we can enjoy satisfying our hunger three times a day throughout our lives with no downside, who can belittle enjoying a cigarette twenty times a day throughout our lives, also with no downside? A closer examination reveals that the similarity is a subtle illusion. In reality the two pastimes are diametrically opposed:

1. Food provides health, energy, happiness, and prolongs our life. Tobacco ruins our health, causes misery and lethargy and shortens our lives.

2. Food tastes good; satisfying your hunger is a genuinely pleasant experience, whereas inhaling cancerous and foul-tasting fumes into your lungs is a decidedly unpleasant experience.

3. Eating doesn't create hunger; on the contrary, it genuinely satisfies it. The fact that it doesn't satisfy it permanently means we can enjoy the pleasure of eating throughout our lives. Far from satisfying the 'little monster', our first cigarette actually creates it. If no further cigarette were smoked, the 'little monster' would die without the person even being aware of its existence. Far from satisfying the 'little monster', each subsequent cigarette simply renews its appetite. The only way to satisfy it is to stop feeding it! Remember: all you actually enjoy when you smoke is attempting to get back to the relaxed state that non-smokers enjoy throughout their lives. Immunity prevents you reaching that relaxed state even for the few minutes that you are partially relieving those withdrawal symptoms.

A good meal at a nice restaurant is a pleasant ritual, however its main purpose is to satisfy a natural hunger at a certain time of the day, and it would be unpleasant if you weren't able to satisfy that hunger. There are parallels with smoking. The gold lighters, the glossy packaging are just like silver snuff-boxes, designed to make a filthy, disgusting 'habit' appear to be glamorous. The whole smoking ritual is designed for one object alone: to try to satisfy that 'little monster'. That's why we have to light the cigarette, that's why we have to stick it in our mouths and that's why we breathe the filth into our lungs:

JUST TO GET THE NICOTINE

Some smokers find it difficult to accept that the only pleasure any smoker gets from lighting a cigarette is the partial and illusory relief of withdrawal symptoms. In case it is not absolutely clear, you do actually feel less tense, more relaxed, less bored and more able to concentrate than you did before you lit up. That is not illusion but real. The illusion is that each cigarette relieves rather than causes the situation. The phenomenon of snuff-taking will help you to see cigarette smoking in its true light.

You are probably aware that snuff is simply powdered tobacco and was the most common form of nicotine addiction prior to the mass production of cigarettes. It is difficult to believe nowadays that it too was once regarded as a highly sociable pastime. Why do cocaine addicts sniff cocaine? Do you believe that they enjoy it purely because it is pleasant to sniff foreign substances up one's nostrils, or do you believe they do it to obtain the effects of the drug? Just as smokers who don't understand the true reasons they smoke create excuses that sound perfectly reasonable (until you examine them closely), so snuff-takers would invent similar excuses. The true reason why any smoker continues to smoke is to end the empty, insecure feeling that the previous cigarette created.

Incidentally, if you harbour illusions about switching to roll-ups, small cigars or even a pipe, forget it! Just because details of the nicotine content are not given on cigar products, this doesn't mean they don't contain nicotine. For convenience I frequently refer just to cigarettes. In case it is not already clear, the term cigarettes should include any item that contains nicotine, including snuff, chewing tobacco, cigars, cigarillos and nicotine gum, patches and sprays. Get it clearly out of your lungs and into your head: you don't become addicted to nicotine because you smoke – you only smoke because you are addicted to nicotine!

It is important to realize that, like a hunger for food, the 'little monster' is actually a physiological reaction. Obviously it isn't a separate organism like a tapeworm, but the effect is exactly the same. It will help you to start thinking of it as an actual living monster that feeds on nicotine. As it grows it creates more discomfort and the uneasy feeling you experience all the time. You created it with the first cigarette and you've been feeding it ever since. Once we've removed the brainwashing, you are going to starve it. Be clear, it won't be like starving a tapeworm of food; that also involves starving yourself for a period. You will only be starving the 'little nicotine monster', not yourself. In the process you will have the added pleasure of no longer having to poison yourself.

Before we move on, there are some important points to establish about nicotine addiction. Although nicotine is the most powerful addictive drug known to mankind, it only relates to the speed in which it traps its victims. The beautiful truth is:

NO SMOKER IS EVER BADLY ADDICTED TO NICOTINE

The term 'nicotine addiction' is in fact a misnomer. It is true that the almost imperceptible physical withdrawal acts as a catalyst to fool us into believing that we get some genuine support or pleasure from smoking. But it is the illusion that hooks us, not the nicotine itself. Remove the brainwashing and you automatically remove the addiction.

Did I mention that the cycle was never-ending? That's only if you continue to feed the 'little monster'. You have no doubt heard that every cigarette takes five minutes off your life and that it takes ten years for the effects to leave your body. These reports are true, but only if you continue to smoke or have contracted a terminal disease. Provided you haven't already done that, you can regain 99 percent of those lost minutes. True, the effects of smoking never disappear completely (there are traces even in non-smokers who come into contact with smokers), but most of it leaves your body within a few weeks.

When we subject our traditional beliefs to closer scrutiny, the established facts are honeycombed with contradictions and paradoxes. If we apply the same level of scrutiny to 'my contention' – that our friendly, sociable pastime of smoking amounts to nothing more than inhaling lethal fumes into our lungs in a vain attempt to remove the empty, insecure feeling that the first cigarette created – then we find that the mysteries, contradictions and paradoxes disappear.

If you analyse your own smoking and observe other smokers, it soon becomes obvious that it is not so much that smokers enjoy smoking cigarettes – they cannot enjoy what would otherwise be a pleasant occasion without them. This might appear to be the same thing, but it isn't. Get it clearly into your mind that you are simply stopping smoking:

YOU DON'T HAVE TO STOP LIVING

I would like you to stop, but not because smoking is a filthy, disgusting addiction that is ruining your health and wealth and depriving you of your freedom, or because it is causing distress to your family. I want you to stop for a purely selfish reason:

YOU WILL ENJOY LIFE SO MUCH MORE

It is true that while you believe that life cannot be enjoyed or stress handled without a cigarette, and that it is almost impossible to 'give up', you might well be prepared to die rather than do so. Almost 5,000,000 smokers take this option every year. The fact is they have no option. They die rather than 'give up' because they don't know how to escape. The beautiful truth is that the physical withdrawal from nicotine is almost imperceptible and gets no worse when you put out your final cigarette. It is the illusions that cause the torture. Fortunately, we can remove the brainwashing before you put out your final cigarette. When you do so, provided you have followed all the instructions, you will already be a happy non-smoker. So, let's get on and do just that. Incidentally, would you even bother to stop if you were one of those:

HAPPY CASUAL SMOKERS?

14 *Happy Casual Smokers*

Heavy smokers find it almost impossible to believe that there is no such being as a happy casual smoker. If you are a casual smoker yourself, you won't be a happy one. If you were happy to be a casual smoker, you wouldn't be reading this book. All smokers have to lie to themselves and to other people. Because they are usually honest, upright citizens in other matters, they are also people we respect, and so we believe their lies. It takes only a cursory examination to explode the myth they have constructed around themselves.

Why should heavy smokers envy casual smokers? When I was a golf fanatic playing three times a week, I didn't envy the poor sap who could play only once a week. I envied professional golfers who could spend their whole lives playing golf. And if heavy smokers envy casual smokers so much, why don't they become casual smokers themselves?

A casual smoker will typically say something like: 'I can take them or leave them. Sometimes I'll go a whole week/month/six months/year without a cigarette.' You think: 'You lucky so and so, I wish I could do that.' But if they genuinely enjoy the taste of a cigarette after a meal or when answering the phone, why on earth would they want to go a whole week without it? If they could genuinely take or leave cigarettes, only a fool would actually take them. After all, everyone knows that smoking is highly addictive, expensive and the No. 1 killer in the Western world. Surely only a complete fool would experiment with something like that, unless, of course, they were actually hooked. I assure you that I can take or leave heroin. I might convince you of the truth of this statement if I never take the drug. I'd be insulting your intelligence if I said,

'I can take it or leave it. Sometimes I'll go a whole week without a shot'!

But have you considered why any smoker would say something like, 'I can take them or leave them. Sometimes I'll go a whole week without a cigarette.'? If I said to you, 'I can go a whole week without carrots and it doesn't worry me', wouldn't you be thinking, 'So what! So can I. Why the need to say it, let alone brag about it?' Anybody who takes heroin, no matter how infrequently, is not a 'user' but an addict. Exactly the same applies to smokers. Remember, we are talking about DEVASTATION. No one would take that drug if they could genuinely leave it.

When casual smokers say something like, 'I can take them or leave them. Sometimes I'll go a whole week without a cigarette', they are trying to convince you and themselves that they do not have a smoking problem. In reality they are admitting to you, if not to themselves, the complete opposite. If they had no problem, there would be no need to make the statement. It is invariably made in a bragging tone. That's because there's a genuine reason for bragging: they have disciplined themselves not to smoke for a whole week.

If you have ever made a successful attempt to cut down, you might remember the self-righteous feeling of those first few days. You have achieved the heavy smoker's dream of paradise: your level of smoking is so low that you no longer have to worry about the expense or of contracting one of those horrific diseases associated with smoking. At the same time, you don't have to 'give up' completely. You believe you have the best of all worlds.

A typical example involves Mary, a young housewife who sought my help. She was trying to stop by cutting down. She had been smoking forty-a-day. One afternoon she screwed up her packet of cigarettes in disgust, and threw it into the trash can. An hour later, she was wading through the potato peelings trying to find a cigarette. The next day she experienced the same revulsion to smoking. She was an intelligent woman and wasn't going to make the same mistake again, so she smeared mustard over the cigarettes before banishing them to the trash can. An hour later she was scraping potato peelings and mustard from those cigarettes. Most smokers have gone through a similar experience in their lives, yet some still insist they smoke only for the marvellous taste.

Mary decided that there was no way she could go through 'cold turkey'. She decided she'd have to ease herself off them. She reasoned, 'I'm smoking forty-a-day. If I cut out just one cigarette each day, that shouldn't take too much willpower. In fact I probably won't even notice it, and provided I stick to my plan, I must end up a non-smoker.'

We've probably all tried variations of this process at one or more times in our smoking lives. It sounds perfectly logical. After about six weeks Mary reached the stage where she was down to just one cigarette a day. The trouble was she couldn't bring herself to cut out that last cigarette. She went another three months smoking just one cigarette a day, then she sought my help. This is how she described her life:

'I'd get my husband off to work and the children off to school. I would sit down and take that cigarette out of the packet, then put it back, thinking I'll do the washing-up first.' After she had finished the washing-up, Mary would repeat the process with the ironing. All day she would be dangling the cigarette like a carrot under her own nose, but she wasn't even kidding herself. She knew that she wasn't going to smoke that cigarette until just before her children came home from school. Then she would sit down and smoke it.

Having craved it all day, can you imagine how enjoyable that cigarette must have seemed to her, and what she had to suffer to obtain that illusory pleasure? You might argue that the pleasure was real. Not so, the cigarette tasted just as bad as it always did. Her pleasure was just the ending of the misery of the craving. If that cigarette had actually ended the misery, I would accept that the pleasure was real. Far from ending it, that cigarette simply caused her to suffer the same misery until she sought my help.

Supposing you had met Mary during the three months she was on one-a-day. Just imagine the willpower and effort she had exerted to get free of the filthy weed. Do you think she made that effort because she wanted to be a smoker, or because she desperately wanted to free herself? If you had enquired how she was getting on during those months (and bear in mind that at this stage she thinks she is succeeding), what do you think her reply would have been? Would it have been, 'Oh, I know that I am wasting my time. Those cigarettes are so gorgeous, I don't even know why I am bothering to go through this trauma.' Or do you think she would have said, 'I'm doing great! Now I need only one cigarette a day!' Your natural reaction would be to envy her. In fact, you should pity her. Envying a casual smoker is equivalent to envying someone who is forced to spend the rest of their life on a permanent diet, with the added disadvantage that the diet is not of food but poison.

Let's now look at Mary's true position. In her logical mind, she was just one cigarette away from being a non-smoker. But for twenty-three hours of every day she was dominated mentally by the thought of the next cigarette, and physically she was suffering, too. The only pleasure in smoking is ending the aggravation of the body craving nicotine. Just like a hunger for food, the longer you suffer it the more marvellous it will seem when you relieve the suffering. Mary wasn't removing her illusory dependence on nicotine, but simply ingraining in her mind that the only precious thing on earth is a cigarette.

If you've ever tried cutting down in any of its various forms, you will know this approach only works for a short period. Some people tell me they have actually succeeded in 'giving up' completely by a gradual cutting down process. Incredibly, many are actually smoking as they explain to me how they did it, and others are chewing nicotine gum! If any smoker has actually succeeded in giving up smoking by weaning themselves off cigarettes gradually, I take my hat off to them. They must have phenomenal willpower. At the same time I can only pity them for the torture they must have inflicted upon themselves.

Why do we believe that it is possible to cut down, either on a permanent basis, or as a stepping stone to 'giving up' permanently? Because with the knowledge we possess it is logical to believe so.

We know several of these happy casual smokers. If they can do it, why not us? After all, during the many years between learning to inhale without feeling sick and before you reached the stage where you got into the habit of smoking excessively, you were one of these happy casual smokers. Or were you? Take a moment to reflect on those years.

Of the thousands of cigarettes that you must have smoked, how many of them can you actually remember smoking? How often can you remember inhaling deeply and thinking, 'This is one gorgeous experience.' Can you remember once thinking to yourself, 'I'm so pleased I took up smoking. I'm so lucky to be a smoker.' Or did you find yourself just drifting into it like every other smoker, blocking your mind to the reality with a vague promise that you would 'give up' one day, when the time was right?

Let's consider the start of Emma Freud's introduction:

'The only thing in my life I've ever really regretted was the day, aged fourteen, when I smoked my first cigarette. Twelve years later, I was smoking twenty a day and loved it, actually relished it, but was terrified about what it was doing to my health.'

The tug-of-war clearly existed. If taking up smoking was indeed the only thing in her life that she regretted, one would assume that the bad side of smoking far outweighed the good. She makes it quite clear what caused the bad side, but makes no attempt to explain why she loved and truly relished smoking. Amazingly, all smokers have this problem, whatever their age or how much they smoke. All some youngsters can come up with is, 'It makes me feel dizzy!' Ask them if they are really prepared to spend tens of thousands and risk awful diseases just to make themselves feel dizzy, when they can achieve exactly the same effect by closing their eyes and spinning around, and not surprisingly they feel somewhat foolish.

Bear in mind that Emma wrote that introduction several months after she stopped smoking, and she clearly still believed she had actually loved and relished smoking. This alone would explain why she got hooked again. Obviously she hadn't removed that particular piece of the brainwashing!

It's human nature that we tend to forget the bad times in our lives and remember the good particularly fondly. Hence the expression 'the good old days': when you could hire a limousine to a classy restaurant, eat a meal that actually tasted like food, see the best show in town and still have money in your wallet at the end of the evening. We tend to overlook the fact that many people didn't have a job, let alone any money and that the majority had to use an outside toilet in winter and had no hot running water.

However, when we look back on our smoking lives, it is only the bad times that we are able to recall. That's why most of us can remember the experience of our first experimental cigarettes; not because they were so marvellous, but because they were foul. We all have memories of searching for an all-night gas station, because we get into a panic without cigarettes. Most of us think that the cigarette after a meal is very special, but of all the thousands of meals you've had, can you remember smoking a single one of them? But you'll remember those meals that were ruined because you weren't allowed to smoke. The girl at the party will never forget the panic of losing one of her last two cigarettes; and Mary will never forget the indignity of wiping mustard from those cigarettes and hating herself for being a slave to nicotine.

If you believe that you smoke at the level you do because you got into the habit of smoking at that level, then it is logical to assume that it's possible to reverse the process. In other words, if you can discipline yourself to gradually smoke less, soon it will become a habit to smoke less and you won't even want to smoke more. Continue the process, and it will soon become a habit not to need or want a cigarette at all. It's so simple and obvious. So why doesn't it work? Why are so many smokers who have actually succeeded in 'giving up' when using a 'willpower' method still craving for occasional cigarettes years after smoking what they hoped would be their last cigarette? And why do so many of them get hooked again?

BECAUSE SMOKING ISN'T HABIT
BUT NICOTINE ADDICTION

We know that cutting down doesn't work. If it did we would all be either casual smokers or ex-smokers. Once you understand the true nature of the trap, you will see clearly that attempts to cut down or to control the level that you smoke ingrains into your brain the idea that you cannot enjoy life or cope with stress without a cigarette.

Imagine the 'little monster' as an almost imperceptible 'itch'. What is the natural course of action if you have an 'itch'? That's right: to scratch it. Perhaps you agree with my wife Joyce that scratching only makes it worse. You may both be right. Even if I make a mosquito bite bleed and it lasts for a month, I would rather scratch it than exercise the necessary discipline to leave it alone. The equivalent as regards smoking is to light a cigarette. As soon as you do, you get relief, but you're not aware this relief will be only temporary.

Allow me to digress for a moment. It was once common for tobacco manufacturers to advertise their brands as 'satisfying' or as 'giving satisfaction'. It doesn't take a genius to deduce that it is not possible to satisfy a given situation without a previous state of dissatisfaction.

Let's examine a few examples. We satisfy a sexual desire, a hunger or a thirst. But you won't satisfy a sexual desire by eating or a thirst by smoking a cigarette. The only aggravation that a cigarette appears to satisfy is the nicotine 'itch', although as I have explained, the relief is only temporary because nicotine is responsible for causing the itch in the first place. Non-smokers don't suffer from this particular aggravation.

When we start to smoke, there tend to be long periods between scratching the 'itch' and its recurrence. But it's not long before we are buying our own cigarettes, smoking on a regular basis rather than just on social occasions, and getting that panic feeling if we don't have cigarettes on us. These changes don't come about because we get into the habit; it is the nature of the beast. As immunity to the relief sets in, the 'itch' becomes permanent, and the natural tendency is to scratch it permanently. In other words: to chain-smoke.

So why don't we all quickly become chain-smokers? Because you need very strong lungs to chain-smoke, believe me. Many smokers cannot physically cope with more than five to ten cigarettes a day. Many others are casual smokers because they cannot afford to smoke more. The vast majority of the minority who don't get hooked in the first place aren't non-smokers because they are more intelligent. It's simply that they couldn't cope with the poisonous effects, or couldn't afford the learning process, or were lucky enough to be in a circle of friends who, for whatever reason, hadn't fallen into the trap.

There are several reasons why nowadays many women are casual smokers, and they all involve feelings of guilt, self-despising and the use of massive self-discipline. A common reason for limiting their intake is so they can set an example to their children and grandchildren. Christine's case is typical and amusing, but also filled with pity:

'I already felt guilty that I was setting a bad example to my daughter, Sarah. When she came home from school and started lecturing me about the evils of smoking and how she was terrified that I would die, I made a determined effort to "give up". It was fine to begin with and I felt so proud of myself. I really thought I had kicked it, then stupidly, after I had put Sarah safely to bed one night, I thought I had earned a little reward. Surely just one cigarette couldn't do any harm. Needless to say it became a regular habit and soon the one became several. To be honest I was chain-smoking every evening. It all came to a head on this particular evening when Sarah wouldn't settle. I left her bedroom in a temper. I knew it wasn't really her fault but I couldn't wait any longer for a cigarette. No sooner had I lit up and started the washing-up than a little voice behind me said: "You aren't smoking are you, Mommy?" I managed to flick the cigarette under the tap, turned around and said: "Of course not, darling." She had tears running down her cheeks. I burst out crying too. I'd lied to my daughter. I felt so wretched but, can you believe it, I actually lit another cigarette in front of her. I loathe myself, but not only haven't I stopped, I'm practically chain-smoking all day. Please, please, can you help me?'

I'm happy to confirm that I was able to. But again, if you had spoken to Christine when she was only smoking one cigarette each evening, she would have convinced you that she was a genuinely happy, casual smoker. And she was. But because of the nature of the beast:

IT COULDN'T LAST

Many smokers discipline themselves not to smoke in various situations: in the car, the house or bedroom. Many young smokers won't smoke in front of their parents. Smoking isn't about individual cigarettes, though. Smoking is a lifetime's chain of nicotine leaving the body and creating that empty, insecure feeling. Take a closer look at the 'I can take it or leave it' smokers. Notice how restless they become when they haven't had a cigarette for a period, and how quickly they find an excuse to have a sneaky puff. See the lighting up of a cigarette not as relieving that 'itch', but as simply replacing the nicotine. Observe how quickly the cigarette burns and how the 'itch' returns the moment it is put out. See the whole tug-of-war as it really is: on one side a permanent 'itch' with an accompanying desire to scratch it permanently. On the other side there are powerful reasons for wishing that you didn't need to scratch it at all.

Cutting down or casual smoking – which amount to the same thing – cannot work, because scratching the 'itch' is the only pleasure any smoker ever gets from smoking. The more you scratch it, the more immune you become to the relief, which makes you want to chain-smoke. But the more you smoke, the greater is the destruction of your health, wealth, nerves, concentration and courage. What a terrible trap drug addiction is: part of your brain wants you to smoke more, and whenever you do the other part wants you to smoke less.

It never seems to occur to us that we are always in the wrong position. Before you decided to cut down, you lit up whenever you felt the need or desire to. You were obviously unhappy with this situation; why else would you decide to cut down? But in order to cut down, you can no longer light up whenever you want to. Therefore you are simply depriving yourself of certain cigarettes. Do you see what I mean? The more you smoke, the less you want to smoke. The less you smoke, the more you want to smoke. Smokers can never win. I know that you are aware of this, but I want you to understand why and to accept the inevitable. Skiers can glide downhill without using any energy whatsoever. But they soon learn how incredibly difficult it is to ski uphill. Being addicted to a drug is like spending your whole life attempting to ski uphill.

When you cut down, you discipline yourself not to relieve the 'itch' immediately. Just as the longer you wear tight shoes, the greater will be the sense of relief when you finally take them off, so the longer you suffer the 'itch' the greater will be the illusion of pleasure when you finally allow yourself to scratch it. This enhancement of the illusion of pleasure actually has the effect of reducing your desire to stop. You might still argue that the less you smoke the less harm you inflict on your health and wealth, and ask what's so bad about that. Just this:

BECAUSE YOUR DESIRE TO STOP IS ALSO REDUCED, YOU MAKE NO ATTEMPT TO STOP

This is why casual smokers are more hooked than heavy smokers. Of the 'I followed all your instructions but Easyway still didn't work for me' letters I receive, the ones that frustrate me the most are those that include something like: 'However, on the bright side, I'm now only smoking about five-a-day. Before I visited your centre I was smoking forty a day!'

Other 'experts' might be delighted by such news. So why does it frustrate me so? Because it means that these smokers have failed to understand the nature of the trap. If smokers deprive themselves of nicotine for a whole week, they obviously get a tremendous sense of relief when they finally allow themselves to scratch the 'itch'. They would obtain a similar sense of relief if they were finally able to relieve themselves following a week of constipation. But no one would deliberately suffer the constipation just to get the relief.

These attempts to cut down or our failed attempts to stop make us believe there is some pleasure or crutch to be had from smoking. Because we feel deprived and miserable when we aren't allowed to smoke, and that misery ends the moment we do, it seems logical to assume that cigarettes do indeed bring us pleasure. Yet when we are able to light up whenever we want to, there doesn't appear to be any pleasure and we just take for granted whatever smoking gives us. It is a strange pastime that, when we are allowed to do it, we cannot understand what pleasure we are receiving, and wish we didn't have to do it. Only when we aren't allowed to do it, does it appear to be pleasurable.

I make no apologies for repeatedly making the same point. The lifetime's brainwashing is powerful because it consists of illusions that seem viable only because they have been repeated millions of times. If you have suffered the misery of a 'willpower' method of trying to 'give up', it is difficult to imagine that the process of stopping smoking can be immediate, easy and enjoyable. But would you get any feeling of relief from constipation unless you suffered from it?

Would you miss that feeling of relief if you didn't suffer the constipation? Of course not. Is it so difficult to believe that if no 'little monster' or nicotine 'itch' existed, and you didn't need to discipline yourself not to scratch it for a week, there would be no need or desire to relieve it, and even if you did there would be no feeling of relief?

You might be able to check this out for yourself. Have you ever got to the stage where you have 'given up' long enough to feel so certain you've kicked it that you want to take a couple of puffs, just to prove the point? If you've done this, you'll know that not only does it taste bad but it does nothing for you whatsoever. However, it does convince you that you couldn't get hooked again. So a week or so later, you feel confident that you can have just one cigarette without getting hooked again. You've fallen into exactly the same trap that you fell into at the start. Literally millions of smokers have genuinely escaped only to fall back into the same trap.

Remember what we are trying to achieve is a frame of mind so that you have no more need or desire to smoke a single cigarette than you would want to inject yourself with heroin. This is why cutting down cannot work; it increases the illusion of crutch and/ or pleasure. It not only keeps the 'little monster' alive, but actually increases the power of the 'big monster'. This is why all the so-called special cigarettes follow a period of abstinence, like the one after a meal, the first of the day and the one after sex.

The only thing you enjoy when you smoke a cigarette is ending the aggravation of craving it. I'm sure I no longer need to emphasize that more nicotine is the one thing that won't end it.

If you see just one cigarette as some form of support or pleasure, you will see a million cigarettes in the same way. I know some 'experts' will advise you that you only need to resist the temptation of smoking just one cigarette: the next one. And the great evil of this statement is that it is true. What they fail to tell you is that if you see that one cigarette as some sort of support or pleasure, you are going to have to spend the rest of your life resisting it! Who would want to do that?

Cutting down cannot work because the nature of the addiction is to get you wanting to scratch the 'itch' more and more, not less and less. An attempt to cut down is like going on a diet: you have to exercise willpower and discipline to succeed. Does dieting make food appear to be less precious? Of course not. Your whole life turns into an obsession with food. After each meal either you feel guilty because you failed to stick to your diet, or feel hungry and dissatisfied because you did. Cutting down on nicotine means going through life suffering the double-aggravation of the 'itch' itself and not being allowed to scratch it when you want to. Such a situation demands permanent willpower and discipline. You might succeed for a while. Remember though that the process intrinsically increases the desire to smoke and reduces the desire to stop. Even if you had the willpower to stand this situation for the rest of your life, do you really want to go through this misery?

Invariably the discipline and willpower are exhausted, and the poor smoker is left more nervous, more self-despising, more convinced that she is lacking in willpower and that she cannot enjoy life or function without nicotine. It's probably another five years before she'll build up the courage to try again. This is why I get so frustrated when I hear: 'On the bright side, I'm now only smoking about five a day.'

Perhaps you still believe there are some genuinely happy, casual smokers who can go through their whole lives never wanting to smoke more than five-a-day. I would ask you to bear in mind two things. The first relates to the examples I quote. They are just that: examples. However, although no two cases are exactly the same, the basic principles are. I have personally helped many thousands of smokers. There is now a network of Easyway centres throughout the world, and regular consultations with and between our therapists confirm my findings. Remember, too, that when these smokers seek our help, they no longer have to keep up the pretence that they are in control or are happy to be smokers, casual or otherwise.

The second point relates to smokers themselves. It's not wise to assume that casual smokers are happy just because they tell you they are, or because we've been brainwashed to assume that happy, casual smokers exist. I can't repeat too often that many smokers will tell you how much they enjoy being smokers, but you try to find just one smoking parent who encourages their children to smoke. This goes for happy, casual smoking parents, too. Talk to these happy, casual smokers. Talk to them privately and you will find that many will admit that they would rather be non-smokers. It doesn't take much probing to realize that the others are hiding behind a shield based on fear. Let me tell you about Deirdre. Her case is typical.

She phoned the centre to demand an individual appointment. It was immediately apparent that she knew what she wanted and was used to getting it. I explained that I was giving group therapy for ten hours a day, seven days a week and that, unless and until the situation eased, I just hadn't got time for anything other than group sessions. Her response was that money wasn't a problem. I was somewhat piqued. I don't know about you, but while I accept that everyone has their price, people who assume I'll do anything for money cause the hairs on the back of my neck to rise. I told her that money wasn't the issue and it was, as I had already explained, just a question of my time, which she was now wasting. When she finally understood, she burst into tears.

The tears were genuine. They were caused by the same evil that has reduced millions of otherwise strong, happy, healthy individuals, both male and female and including myself, to tears of desperation: slavery to nicotine.

Perhaps you find nothing unusual about this. But Deirdre had been smoking for twelve years during which time she had never smoked more than two cigarettes a day. Her state was every heavy smoker's vision of paradise. How many of them would believe that just smoking two cigarettes a day could reduce her to a state of despair?

Had she contracted lung cancer or some other fatal disease? On the contrary, she was a physical fitness fanatic and incredibly healthy. However, lung cancer did play a part in her anxiety; both her parents had died from lung cancer before she fell into the trap. Like me, she had a great fear of smoking before she became hooked. She too had eventually given in to the immense social pressure, tried an experimental cigarette, and found it repulsive. Unlike me, who capitulated to chain-smoking in no time at all, Deirdre resisted. But she had the same schizophrenia as every other smoker. Like a hunger for food, the longer you crave a cigarette, the more precious it will appear when you finally satisfy that craving. And, of course, the less you smoke, the less you cripple your health and your pocket, and the less you need to stop.

Because both her parents died from lung cancer, Deirdre concluded that she must have a congenital flaw. My brother has the same morbid fear of cancer, because both our sister and father died from cancer in their mid-fifties. It's incredible that the human race has survived hundreds of thousands of years without cancer. In 1900 only one in fifty UK citizens died from cancer. Today it's one in four. Why do we blame our parents or the incredible intelligence that designed us? If you were stupid enough to pour salt water over your car on a daily basis, would you blame the manufacturer for its being riddled with rust? We poison our lungs, our food, our rivers and the very air that we breathe on an hourly basis, and then spend billions of pounds searching for cures. Yet the cures are so simple and obvious. Obliterate the conditions that cause these diseases. I could obliterate smoking and all drug addiction with just one billionth of those funds.

Deirdre's parents died for exactly the same reason as my sister and father: they were heavy smokers. Deirdre was terrified of increasing her intake lest she contract lung cancer, like her parents. But she was only smoking two cigarettes a day. Surely it should have been easy to cut those out? Yes, that is what we've been brainwashed to believe. This is the reason we can't understand why our children continue to dabble, why they can't see that they might get hooked. But it's us that can't see. We can't even prevent our children and grandchildren from falling into the trap.

Deirdre's fear of cancer inspired her to exercise the necessary willpower and discipline to restrict her smoking to just two cigarettes a day. If you've got a permanent 'itch' but only allow yourself to scratch it twice a day, that takes enormous willpower and discipline. But let me remind you: the smoker's 'itch' is a feeling of emptiness, insecurity and lack of courage and confidence. The longer you suffer it, the more it wears down your resistance and the more precious that little 'friend' and crutch appears when you light up. If you are ever tempted to envy a casual smoker again, remember they spend the bulk of their lives suffering that empty, insecure feeling. Do you really believe that Deirdre was one of those happy, casual smokers? If she was, why did she seek my help? Throughout those twelve years she spent only twenty minutes of each day partially relieving the 'itch' and over twenty-three hours suffering it. What's the longest you've managed to last in an attempt to cut down, or to become a casual smoker (which amounts to the same thing)?

How do you think Deirdre appeared to her non-smoking friends and colleagues? Deirdre was so ashamed of herself that she could never bring herself to smoke in front of them. That's because she thought they would be thinking things like, 'I can't understand her. She's obviously very strong-willed and highly intelligent. If she smokes only occasionally, she can't be badly hooked, so why does she bother? Surely she can't be oblivious to the smell on her breath, hair and clothes?'

I've absolutely no doubt that her smoking friends and colleagues were actually envious of her. Of course, she didn't tell them of the nightmare she was going through. She didn't want them to realize how stupid and weak she felt, any more than any other drug addict wants to. Can you imagine the willpower and discipline it took to keep up the pretence for twelve years? Is it so difficult to understand how such a strong-willed, self-sufficient and intelligent woman was reduced to pleading for my help when she must dearly have wanted to hang-up on me? It was no credit to me, but I'm so pleased that she didn't. It is simply more evidence of how the evil 'weed' destroys its victims, not just physically but also mentally.

Deirdre is probably the strongest-willed person I have ever met. In the next chapter we will explode the myth that smokers who have failed to stop are lacking in willpower. In particular, we will explode the myth that the reason there are more women smoking than men, and more young girls getting hooked than boys, is because women are in general weaker, less intelligent, more ruled by emotion than logic and less strong-willed than men.

However, before we do so, we need to dispel one more myth about casual smokers. Let's now consider the type of casual smoker that other smokers probably envy most of all, the 'I don't find "giving up" a problem, I can do it whenever I want to' type.

Of course we envy such smokers. But if I tried to sell you Aladdin's lamp, would you just take my word that it indeed had 'magical' properties? It doesn't take a Sherlock Holmes to deduce that smokers who can 'give up' whenever they want to just don't exist. To start with, it's a contradiction in terms; if they have truly 'given up', they wouldn't have started again once let alone several times. And why would they want to 'give up'? After all, no one forces us to 'give up' any more than they can force us to smoke in the first place. So, isn't it obvious? No smoker would 'give up' unless they didn't enjoy being a smoker. And when they do 'give up', why on earth do they start again? The answer is equally obvious: they don't enjoy being non-smokers either.

We believe such smokers get the best of both worlds. Please don't envy them. Like every other smoker, heavy, casual or otherwise, they actually get the worst of all worlds: during the periods they are smokers, they wish they were non-smokers. Why else would they 'give up'? And during their non-smoking phases they feel deprived and miserable. Why else would they start again?

Never forget that although all smokers are different, they are all hooked on the same drug. It's not a case of one man's food is another man's poison. This particular drug is poisonous to all living creatures. To each and every one of them it is undiluted:

DEVASTATION

I'm sure that message has got home to you. But perhaps you are still worried by the thought that you too will be like the stoppers and starters: miserable whether you smoke or not. It is a common belief: once a smoker, always a smoker. In other words, no matter how many years you've 'given up', an ex-smoker will never feel the same as someone who never fell into the trap. Of course, this is true for the majority of ex-smokers, because with a 'willpower' method you do believe that you have given up a genuine support or pleasure.

However, with Easyway you actually feel better than a non-smoker. Many non-smokers, although they are happy to be non-smokers, actually believe that they are missing out. After all, they are subjected to the massive brainwashing, and why would any of us be tempted to try those first experimental cigarettes unless we suspected that there was some pleasure or support? Their attitude tends to be, what you've never had you don't miss. With Easyway you first see quitting smoking as it really is:

WAKING FROM A FRIGHTENING NIGHTMARE

Now let's explode one of the most powerful and damaging of all the myths, that:

IT TAKES WILLPOWER TO STOP

15 *It Takes Willpower To Stop*

So powerful is this particular myth that the controllers of TV and radio advertising won't allow a stop smoking commercial to be broadcast unless it includes a statement to the effect that the aid will only work in conjunction with the smoker's own willpower. Consider the conversation I had with an official of the Advertising Standards Authority (ASA), following his perusal of an advert I had submitted.

ASA: 'I regret that I cannot allow your advert in its present form. You need to include a statement to the effect that your method will only work in conjunction with the smoker's own willpower.'

Me: 'One of the cornerstones of Easyway is that it doesn't require the use of willpower.'

ASA: 'Look sir, there is no problem here, all you need to do is make a slight amendment to the effect that it does.'

Me: 'But I understood that the only purpose of ASA is to protect the public from false or misleading statements.'

ASA: 'Sure' [spoken rather smugly].

Me: 'So how can you possibly justify advising me to tell a lie?'

ASA: [Smugness beginning to be replaced by confusion] 'It's not a lie. It's not possible to give up smoking without using willpower!'

Me: 'Are you an expert on the subject?'

ASA: 'I know nothing about it.'

Me: 'Are you aware that I'm considered by many to be the world's leading expert on the subject?'

ASA: 'I'm aware of your reputation, but everyone knows that it takes willpower to give up smoking.'

Me: 'Tell me, if you didn't want to get on a No. 9 bus, would you need willpower not to get on it?'

ASA: 'Obviously not.'

Me: 'You must have heard of smokers who suddenly lost the desire to smoke and found it easy to stop. Well, that's how Easyway works. Now, if a smoker has no need or desire to smoke, why should it take willpower not to do so?'

ASA: [last traces of smugness gone, now just confusion and anger] 'Look, I'm trying to be helpful, but a rule is a rule.'

Me: 'But if smokers were able to stop using their own willpower, they wouldn't need the gimmicks that you allow to be advertised. Over 2,000 smokers die from smoking every week in the UK. Every smoker is crying out for a method that is easy and doesn't need willpower. You agree that the ASA's only function is to protect the public. In no way can a rule that prevents smokers from knowing about a method that will help them to stop be described as protecting the public.
'On the contrary ASA is actually aiding and abetting their deaths! The rule is clearly a stupid rule and should be changed.'

ASA: 'I can only agree, but only the doctor who made the rule has the power to change it.'

Another rule prevented me from making contact with this so-called expert or even of being allowed to know his name.

It's not surprising that smokers who fail to stop feel that they are weak-willed jellyfish. We have been subjected to massive brainwashing from birth to the effect that 'giving up' can be very difficult, but with sufficient willpower you can succeed. So when someone like me, who always hated being a smoker, failed umpteen times when using his own willpower, what other explanation was there, other than that I was a weak-willed jellyfish? I certainly believed that to be the case. But why did it only relate to my smoking? Why was I so strong-willed in other aspects of my life? Because 'giving up' smoking has nothing to do with willpower. It is a conflict of wills.

Let's look at some unquestionable facts. Look back at your schooldays when some groups of girls experimented and others didn't. Which girls led the way? Was it the shy, retiring bookworms or the physically strong and dominant? Just open your mind and the facts clearly explode the myths. Who were the role models who helped so many teenage girls fall into the trap? Wasn't it the Elle Macphersons, Joanna Lumleys, Kate Moss's? Did any of them strike you as being weak-willed?

Every year the 'media' declares the second Wednesday in March 'National No Smoking Day'. This is the day every smoker is supposed to decide to 'give up'. Yet every smoker will tell you that it is the one day in the year they will do their utmost to resist such pressure. Just to reinforce the point many will smoke more blatantly and twice as many cigarettes as usual. They resent being patronized by people, no matter how well meaning, who haven't the slightest understanding of the smoker's problems.

In the immediate aftermath of the 11 September terrorist attacks on the United States the authorities announced twenty suspected cases of anthrax in the country, two of which were later confirmed and turned out to be fatal. Twenty unconfirmed cases in the UK were then announced. A national daily newspaper reported that the British had stockpiled no fewer than 50 million antidotes to anthrax. The UK government's expert advice was: 'be careful but don't panic'. Do they think we are complete morons? Do we really need that sort of 'expert' advice? The connection between smoking and lung cancer has been established for nearly half a century. Do they really believe it helps to tell smokers one day a year that smoking is injurious to health, when it's been written on every packet of cigarettes for the last umpteen years?

Why doesn't it dawn on these so-called 'experts' that smokers don't smoke because smoking injures their health, and that the real challenge is to remove the reasons that make them continue to smoke. Because these 'experts' don't understand the nature of the nicotine trap, let alone the solution. All smokers instinctively know that smoking isn't exactly conducive to good health. However, let's use those cancer scares to establish once and for all that a smoker's inability to stop has nothing to do with lack of willpower, but a conflict of wills.

There can be no doubt whatsoever that, while we might be influenced by peer pressure, advertising and other brainwashing to fall into the trap and to remain in it, no one can force us either to smoke a cigarette or not to smoke one. It is equally obvious that when we try to 'give up', if we had no desire to light up, quitting would be a simple matter. But we've been brainwashed to believe that smoking gives us some pleasure and/or support. At one end of the see-saw are the 'goodies': the bad effect smoking has on our health and wealth. But hold on, shouldn't these be the 'baddies'? No! This is part of the confusion that the nicotine trap creates in our minds. The belief that smoking supplies some sort of support or pleasure makes you want to continue to smoke, so they are the real 'baddies', particularly as the belief is based on an illusion. The genuine destruction of your health and wealth are forces that make you want to 'give up', so in this context they are the 'goodies'.

But the see-saw isn't static and the respective weights of the 'goodies' and 'baddies' keeps changing. While we have no intention of quitting, we close our minds to the health and wealth aspects and they effectively have no weight. During these periods, if we have no need or desire to light up the 'goodies' still prevail, keeping the 'baddies' high and dry at the top end of the see-saw. However, sooner or later the 'little monster' starts to 'itch'. A desire to light up is now created, the weight of the 'baddies' increases and when the scales are tipped, the 'baddies' swing down and the 'goodies' are raised up. When we light a cigarette, the desire is satisfied and down come the 'goodies'.

However, when we decide to 'give up' we open our minds to the bad effects on our health and wealth. In other words our level of consciousness is raised, substantially increasing the combined weight of the 'goodies' so that even when the 'little monster' signals to the brain: 'I want or need a cigarette', the response is: 'That might well be, but we are now through with all that foolishness and I'm afraid you can't have one.'

Now the 'big monster' comes into play. A slight 'itch' isn't such a problem, provided you can scratch it. But an itch that you can't scratch? That can drive you crazy! It's bad enough if you can't reach it, because you're prevented by some sort of restraint or a plaster cast or if, like me, you are somewhat physically inflexible. How do those mosquitoes find the one square inch on my back that I cannot reach, no matter what miracle of contortion I attempt? The only course of action open to me then is to try rubbing my back against a brick wall or stopping a complete stranger and begging them to scratch the afflicted part for me. Even worse, though, is when the itch is easily accessible to you, but you won't allow yourself to scratch it!

Now, if you have an itch that part of your brain doesn't want you to scratch, it would take an enormous feat of willpower to resist scratching it. But this doesn't mean that, all other things being equal, a strong-willed person will resist longer than a weak-willed person. What cannot be denied is that, regardless of the strength of their respective willpower, both people have a conflict of wills. Supposing the weak-willed person's itch disappears permanently after five minutes and the strong-willed person's 'itch' lasts for six months. It would take enormous willpower to resist scratching a permanent itch for six months. If after the six months the person's resistance, or willpower, or however you want to describe it, was exhausted, and it happened to be the smoker's 'itch', society would conclude that the weak-willed smoker was strong-willed and vice versa. It would conclude wrongly.

A similar tug-of-war, or smoker's schizophrenia, applies to many walks of life. Before the association between smoking and lung cancer was made, most smokers were happy to put up with smoker's cough, asthma, bronchitis and general lethargy, regarding them as a small price to pay for their pleasure and crutch. But the risk of cancer added considerable weight to the 'goodies'. Many smokers decided that the cake was no longer worth the candle and decided to stop. Others argued that the connection hadn't actually been proved, and even if it were true, surely you couldn't spend your life in a plastic bubble protected from all risks. You might step under a truck tomorrow! Were the ones who stopped really being sensible and strong-willed or were they simply panicking and being cowardly? Soldiers who quit the trenches in the First World War because they regarded the whole business as stupidity were shot for being cowards. It takes courage to accept the risk of lung cancer and to resist the pressures to stop that smokers are subjected to nowadays. So are smokers who continue to smoke in spite of those risks and pressures actually being strong-willed?

The evidence suggests that in most cases they are. If you judge the individual smoker's level of willpower not on the basis of whether or not they were able to stop smoking, but on other aspects of their lives, you will find that the smokers who have failed to stop tend to be dominant, strong-willed people. Our most enjoyable cigarettes or, more accurately, the ones we describe as tasting the best, tend to be the ones we have when we are relaxing, like the one after a meal or when we are socializing, situations in which the pleasure quotient is already pretty high. But the cigarettes that make it difficult for us to 'give up' are the ones we need, or the ones we cannot survive without; for example, when we have to concentrate or are under stress. Dominant, strong-willed people tend to take on more responsibility and stress is part and parcel of their lives. Cigarettes go with their lifestyle.

Now is a convenient time to explain another myth. It is true that your favourite brand appears to taste better than other brands.

This is because you have trained your lungs to become partially immune to the particular concoction of poisons contained in your particular brand. But have you noticed how smokers whose brand isn't available for some reason will smoke old rope rather than abstain? Millions of smokers have deliberately switched brands or to roll-ups, cigars or pipes in the hope that this will help them to 'give up', cut down or save money. It isn't long before the new brand becomes their favourite and their previous favourite becomes offensive, providing further proof that taste or enjoyment has nothing to do with smoking – it's just the nicotine we are after.

Clever advertising using attractive role models has convinced some smokers that the ritual of smoking, or smoking purely for smoking's sake, is pleasurable and that the nicotine and poisons are an unfortunate side effect.

If only someone could invent a clean cigarette, smokers sometimes sigh. Someone has, and their invention has been around for years: herbal cigarettes. If you've tried them, you'll know that no matter how long you persevere, you will never achieve even the illusion of pleasure by smoking them. Smoking herbal cigarettes is just like breathing bad fumes into your lungs. The reason that they'll never give you the illusion of enjoyment is that they contain no nicotine. Smoking tobacco also consists purely of inhaling bad fumes into your lungs, but if it weren't for the nicotine there wouldn't be an illusion of a crutch or pleasure.

So why does the identical cigarette out of the same packet appear to taste marvellous after a meal, but bad if it's the first cigarette after the New Year's party? Because it's not the smoking of the cigarette itself that's important, but the time at which you scratch the 'itch'. After a meal, you have already satisfied two aggravations: your hunger and thirst, so you feel relaxed. The cigarette after the evening meal tends to taste better than the one you smoke after breakfast or lunch because work for the day is over and you feel entitled to unwind and relax. This is especially so if the meal you are having is at a restaurant, because if you are a housewife, work for the day isn't usually over at dinner-time. On the contrary, you are not only the chef, but the waitress and chief dishwasher. A meal at a restaurant is special and more relaxing, and if you are having it with friends or in the company of someone special, you are not bored. If the meal is to celebrate some special occasion, such as a wedding, a birthday or Christmas, you feel even more happy and relaxed. No doubt you do have other aggravations in your life, but for those few hours they are forgotten, and your feeling of complete bliss can actually be enhanced because you have other problems. In other words, at such times, you are on a complete and utter 'high'.

But at such times don't you discreetly slip off that special pair of shoes? They might complement the rest of your outfit to perfection, but why oh why are such shoes always available in every size except yours? It's just another classic example of Murphy's law. The point is that it's impossible to enjoy complete and utter bliss while wearing tight shoes. It's exactly the same if you happen to be addicted to nicotine. It's not so much that smokers enjoy a cigarette after a meal or that it tastes any better than it does at any other time. The point is that unless they are allowed to scratch the 'itch', they do not feel relaxed at all. On the contrary, if they are not allowed to smoke, they actually feel deprived and miserable. The difference between smoking and not smoking at such a time is not just a slight buzz, but the difference between paradise and purgatory. That's why the cigarette after a meal or a drink appears to taste better.

In fact the whole question of willpower is irrelevant.

You could argue that the smokers who stopped when the lung cancer connection was established did so because they were being sensible and strong-willed. You could also argue that they were scared and weak-willed. It makes no difference, either way it increased the weight of the 'goodies'. With many smokers the risk was enough to tip the balance permanently. With me, and many others, it wasn't. The problem is, the moment you attempt to 'give up', the combined weight of the 'goodies' tends to decrease. You are no longer risking awful diseases. The cough, asthma and bronchitis soon disappear. You are no longer burning your money or despising yourself for being a slave to nicotine. In other words: all the powerful forces that made you want to 'give up' in the first place are rapidly disappearing. The facts don't actually change, but your perception of them does and it's your perception that is important in the conflict of wills.

While the combined weight of the 'goodies' is decreasing, on the other side of the see-saw the weight of the 'baddies' is increasing. When you smoked the cost drained your finances. Now you have money in your pocket again and can afford the occasional packet of cigarettes. But, most important of all, when you 'give up', you believe that you have made a genuine sacrifice: you've had to resist scratching the 'itch' for a few days, all of which is making you feel deprived and miserable. We all know in our rational minds that the combined weight of the 'goodies', or reasons for being a non-smoker, far exceeds the combined weight of the 'baddies'. The problem is it takes just one weak, stupid, drunken or unguarded moment in our lives when the 'baddies' appear to outweigh the 'goodies' for us to light up again. Just one cigarette and, because it's drug addiction, we find ourselves back in the trap we fell into in the first place.

So stop seeing smokers as jelly-fish and a failure to stop as being due to lack of willpower. See it as it really is: a conflict of wills in which the strength of the combatants is continually varying. Now look at the true position: that smoking not only doesn't confer any pleasure or crutch whatsoever, but actually destroys your nerves, confidence, courage and ability to concentrate and to relax; that far from relieving boredom and stress, it is a major cause of both. In other words, supposing there was no conflict or confusion, that you could remove all the brainwashing, see smoking as it really is, DEVASTATION, then you would have no need or desire to light a cigarette. If you have no need or desire to smoke, it doesn't take one bit of willpower not to. It is irrelevant whether you are weak-willed or otherwise. Willpower is irrelevant.

If willpower is irrelevant, why have I spent so much time discussing the subject? Because one of the evils of all drug addiction is the ingraining into victims' minds that they have some intrinsic flaw in their physical and/or mental make-up and are dependent on the magic provided by the drug in order to enjoy life or cope with stress. It is obvious that smoking provides us with no physical advantages, nor does it provide pleasure or a crutch. The feeling of weakness, both physical and mental, that smokers experience is caused by the drug and is not inherent in the smokers themselves.

Some smokers can see clearly that nicotine addiction simply creates an illusion of pleasure and/or crutch, are convinced and happy that they will never smoke again, but still feel that something is missing in their lives. This extract of a letter from Fiona is typical:

'I understand and agree with everything you say in Easyway. In fact, I now realise that my smoking was a major cause of my marriage break-up. Let me make it clear that I'm deliriously happy to be a non-smoker and know that I will never smoke again. However, I do have just one problem that I don't seem able to solve. I work in a non-smoking office. I would never smoke in the street and couldn't smoke on the train. I can't remember that first cigarette when I got home being particularly important before the separation, but afterwards it became the fulcrum of my life. I know you say that whenever I think about smoking it must be "isn't it great! I'm free", and that's how I genuinely feel all the time, except when I open the front door to that empty house. I can't help thinking:"If only I could have just one cigarette". Because I know it won't be only one cigarette, I don't have it. But I've been free for six months now. Can you please help me?'

I could sympathize with Fiona, as I'm sure you can. In fact, I could only admire her for resisting the temptation. I'm sure that similar circumstances have caused many smokers to fall into the trap again. I asked her if she felt it would have been a problem had the house not been empty. She was emphatic: it wouldn't. It's really part of a very common syndrome: 'It's my little reward'. This is very important for people with boring or stressful lives. It's easy when you find out that smoking destroys your concentration and nerves, because you won't feel the need to put something in its place. But when you've truly believed that smoking offers a reward, you will feel that you've lost that reward, even though it is illusory.

I say to ex-smokers: 'No problem. You can get exactly the same effect by wearing tight shoes, then whenever you need a little reward, just remove them for a few moments.' They don't see this as a solution; in fact, they think I'm being facetious.

But it does help them to see the true position. Fiona's real problem was going home to a house that contained no companion. Hopefully she has solved that problem now. Thank goodness she had the sense to see that there would be little point in compounding her unhappiness by falling into the trap again and thus creating more problems. The same applies to smokers in other situations where they believe that a cigarette is a little reward. If you can't kid yourself into believing that wearing tight shoes will solve the problem, what's the point of kidding yourself that Western society's No. 1 killer disease will solve the problem? If your lifestyle is boring and stressful, the only real solution is to change it. You'll probably find, as I did, that quitting smoking actually cured the boredom and the stress. Fiona was sensible to realize that a cigarette wouldn't solve the problem. I managed to persuade her that if she could see the sense of that and wasn't going to smoke, there was little point in torturing herself by thinking about cigarettes!

When you stop smoking, you don't need anything to take its place. You could enjoy life and cope with stress before you were tricked into believing that you needed phoney crutches or props. You might well feel genuinely weak and insecure at the moment, even though you are a casual smoker. Remember Deirdre was reduced to tears and she was only smoking two-a-day. Such feelings of weakness and insecurity are compounded by the fact that women smokers are subjected to a heinous form of brainwashing that is not applied to men. This brainwashing would have us all believe that women are not only physically weaker than men, but generally are less intelligent, less logical, more emotional and less able to take responsibility.

It is important when quitting smoking to realize that the feelings of weakness and insecurity are genuine. It is even more important to realize that these feelings are caused by smoking and that if you follow all the instructions, courage and confidence that you had forgotten you had will return in no time at all. I know you will find this difficult to believe if you have ever gone through the torture of a 'willpower' attempt to 'give up'. I assure you that it is true. Now, it's high time we established:

WHICH IS THE STRONGER SEX?

16 *Which Is The Stronger Sex?*

Even today there is an assumption that men are generally physically and mentally stronger than women. It is a 'fact' that for generations we have been conditioned to believe. There is no doubt that in Western society more women than men are now smoking. This trend is also reflected in the numbers of youngsters who fall into the smoking trap. Why should this be so?

The so-called 'experts' somewhat glibly explain it as a consequence of the more intelligent smokers having seen the light and attempting to stop. Those with sufficient willpower manage to succeed, their argument runs, which is an underhand way of saying that generally men are more intelligent and stronger-willed than women. It is not just coincidence that the majority of the 'experts' who make such pronouncements are men.

Now let's look at the facts. We have already established that the dominant and strong-willed representatives of both sexes tend to be the role models who assist the rest of us into the trap. We can't have it both ways. In the bad old days when over 80 percent of adult males smoked, men who didn't smoke were regarded as sissies. There happens to be a logical basis for this belief: you need a strong pair of lungs to inhale the filthy fumes and considerable willpower to complete the learning process. The true reason why the other 20 percent managed to evade the trap was not so much that they were more intelligent, but more that they couldn't either physically cope with the poison or afford it.

The 'experts' spend many hours speculating why youngsters fall into the trap. Like every other aspect of nicotine addiction, they would learn so much more by researching the opposite: why other youngsters don't fall into it. So the logical conclusion is that if smokers tend to be physically and mentally stronger than non-smokers, modern woman is stronger than modern man. In truth she always has been!

I have explained the smoker's 'itch': the 'little monster' or desire to light up. I've also referred to the obvious restlessness or discomfort that smokers experience when they wish to scratch the 'itch' but, for whatever reason, aren't able to light up. I call this the smoker's 'twitch': a hand over the mouth, grinding of the jaw, tapping cigarettes, or flicking lighters are all examples. If a friend tells you that she 'must eat', you know she has a genuine need for food and won't be happy until she has satisfied her hunger. You understand the distinction between someone needing food and simply fancying a bite, and accept it. Many non-smokers find it difficult to understand why a smoker would even want a cigarette, let alone need one. But a non-smoker who is involved with a heavy smoker can see clearly that they don't want a cigarette, but need a cigarette. The non-smoker cannot understand why this should be so, but is in no doubt that the smoker is dependent and a slave.

My mother was a non-smoker. Neither of us could understand what we flippantly referred to as the 'dawn chorus': my father, eyes watering, coughing up his lungs. It was blatantly obvious to us that he was receiving no genuine pleasure from smoking. Having watched him die from lung cancer, how it must have pained her to watch me become a smoker, powerless to make me see sense. She did, however, know instinctively the sway that my wife held over me. She said to Joyce: 'Why don't you threaten to leave him if he doesn't give up?' Joyce replied: 'Because he can't give up and would let me leave.' Joyce, also a non-smoker, could no more understand the stupidity than could my mother. She knew how hard I'd tried to stop and had the sense to see that I wasn't smoking because I wanted to, but because I believed that I couldn't enjoy or cope with life without it! I'm ashamed to admit that, as much as I love her, if she had delivered that ultimatum I could not have stopped. This simply illustrates the fear that smoking creates and instils in its victims.

The distinction between 'wanting' and 'needing' a cigarette is very important to smokers themselves. They will willingly admit to needing food or, providing they are not alcoholic, a drink. But they will never admit to needing a cigarette. Because of the social stigma, many of the more considerate smokers make it a rule not to smoke in the car or the house of a non-smoking friend. If that non-smoking friend says: 'If you need a cigarette, it doesn't bother us, feel free to light up in the house', invariably they'll find it necessary to point out that they never need a cigarette but occasionally enjoy one. They will then make a point of not lighting up for an extended period to prove to their friend, and to themselves, that they are in control. It doesn't seem to occur to them that they are simply proving the exact opposite. When they can stand it no longer, they will excuse themselves from the house or restaurant table. If it is again pointed out that their smoking isn't bothering anyone else and that they are welcome to stay, invariably they will refuse on the grounds that they don't wish to be anti-social. It doesn't occur to this smoker that their non-smoking friends would rather have their company, smoke and all, and that depriving them of it is to be truly anti-social.

The sociable cigarettes, like the one after a meal, appear to be the most pleasurable, but we can survive without that illusion. But it's when we are under stress that we really need a cigarette. Intelligent, dominant people tend to have responsible jobs, for various reasons: prestige, higher pay, a requirement for stimulation, etc.

However, we associate responsibility with stress and this is why intelligent, dominant people tend to be heavy smokers. Logically you would expect intelligent, strong-willed smokers to consume less than others. But, as with other aspects of smoking, unless you understand the nature of the trap completely, the facts tend to contradict the logic.

There can be no doubt that women generally have considerably more roles to juggle in their lives than the average man. It's not that long ago that a wife's property rights transferred to her husband on marriage. Indeed at one time the wife herself was considered to be his property. Traditionally women were considered fit only for menial jobs such as housework or, if they had no families of their own, carrying out similar functions for the sick or disabled or the aristocracy. Even aristocratic ladies were regarded as competent only to carry out charitable or social work.

It hurts me at group centres when to the question 'What is your profession?' a woman replies, in an apologetic tone and with a lowering of the head, 'I'm only a housewife.'

Let's take a closer look at the actual functions that 'I'm only a housewife' performs. Allow me to use the one I know best as an example: Joyce. I'm completely absorbed in my quest to see smoking reduced to the same level as that previous form of nicotine addiction, snuff-taking. In order that I have nothing to distract me, Joyce performs 99 percent of all other functions in our lives. She carries out all the traditional housewifely functions, such as washing and ironing, shopping for food and household products, keeping the house clean and tidy, preparing meals, cooking and doing the dishes. She not only buys all my clothes but lays them out for me, because if she didn't I would waste hours prevaricating over what to put on. At one time she looked after the children's needs as well, dealing with upset tummies at all hours of the night and never once complaining. The tasks I've listed probably amount to only a tenth of what I have actually noticed over the years.

I would ask you to ignore my shortcomings and concentrate on Joyce. In addition to being a housewife, she is my partner in the business of helping smokers to stop. She acts as telephonist and receptionist. She pays the bills and keeps the accounts. If we need plumbers or electricians, she organizes them, too. When we travel, she arranges the flights, hotels, currency, car hire, etc. Last, but by no means least, she acts as my adviser, my comforter and my confidence-builder.

She allows me to concentrate all my efforts on just one goal. Frankly I'm incapable of performing more than one function at a time effectively. Occasionally, she might ask me to wire an electric plug or check the oil level in the car. I'm ashamed to admit that on occasions I've been known to react to such requests with suggestions that she attend a course on motor mechanics. I forgot to mention that she does the gardening as well as the housework, and that we employ no gardener or domestic help.

Joyce, in common with most women, can and does perform a thousand and one tasks, and completes them all with great efficiency. It is true that many daily household chores are mundane. Just as someone not equipped to handle responsibility will find that stressful, so an intelligent person completing mundane tasks will find them boring and stressful.

I know that Joyce is highly intelligent, yet unbelievably, she carries out all these tasks cheerfully and never complaining. As her name suggests, she is a joy to be with.

I'm often complimented on my achievements and Joyce sits there nodding her head in agreement, completely oblivious of her own contribution. I don't know who said: 'Behind every great man, you'll find a great woman.' Whoever it was, he got it slightly wrong. He should have said: 'Behind every rather mediocre man, you'll find a great woman.' Joyce didn't make herself a slave to me. She does what she does unselfishly because she loves me and believes in the cause as much as I do. I don't think of her as a typical woman but as the greatest creature that ever lived. But then I'm biased. However, I do believe that our shortcomings and qualities are shared with most other men and women.

Women's liberation has done much to help improve female voting and property rights and been partly able to equalize salaries and job opportunities. Ironically some of these gains have served only to increase the stress in a woman's life. In order to be treated equally in professions that were once regarded as the preserve of men, a woman has to be ten times as good as her male counterpart. Most career women not only have the stress of the career itself, but also the traditional stresses of pregnancy, childbirth, bringing up, feeding, clothing and waiting on the children, including the adult child.

A word of warning, ladies. You might well conclude from what I've been saying that it is more difficult for you to stop smoking, or even that you would be wise to continue to smoke. Not so. All that I am saying is that, whether it's just or otherwise, women tend to have more stress in their lives than men. That being the case, they are more likely to fall into the smoking trap and to remain in it. Get it clearly into your mind: smoking doesn't relieve stress. It causes it. Indeed, for most smokers nicotine addiction is not only the major cause of their stress, but it's what causes so many other aspects of their lives to appear stressful.

I'm not just referring to the effect that the cumulative poisoning and financial cost has on our physical and mental health, energy and self-respect, although all of these factors increase the stress in our lives. I'm also referring to the anxious, empty, insecure feeling that nicotine creates. The effect on smokers is to transform trivial, everyday setbacks, which non-smokers take in their stride, into great traumas. I implied earlier that the only reason I became a chain-smoker was because of the stress created by the fact that I hated my job. The true reason was my addiction to nicotine, which caused me to have the stress in the first place. That is the nature of the beast.

Assume for a moment that cigarettes did relieve stress. You'd expect smokers to be relatively calm and laid-back compared to non-smokers. Is this the reality? Isn't it the smokers who seem to be uptight and restless, particularly when they aren't allowed to smoke? Haven't you found yourself yelling at the kids to go to sleep so you can 'safely' sneak outside for a cigarette? Isn't it the smokers who always need something to do with their hands or something to calm their nerves? If cigarettes do calm their nerves, why do smokers remain so nervous?

Your life will be less stressful once you have stopped smoking. Mother Nature has already equipped you to deal adequately with normal stress. She hasn't equipped you to deal with the evils of smoking, but she has supplied you with adequate warning signs not to smoke.

There are far too many sad aspects to smoking. It is difficult to decide which is the saddest, but high on the list is:

SMOKING DURING PREGNANCY

17 *Smoking During Pregnancy*

This is, without doubt, one of the big No-Nos as far as society is concerned. There is no comparable situation I can think of in which smokers are made to feel so bad about themselves. Interestingly smokers who are pregnant agree wholeheartedly with their accusers and will contribute to the opprobrium heaped upon them. The many letters I receive from smoking mothers are full of self-blame and self-loathing. The women condemn themselves for setting a bad example to their children and for running the risk of leaving them motherless. Those who swore that they would 'give up' if ever they became pregnant feel even worse about themselves. This extract of a letter from Jean is an extreme example:

'It's ironic that during the first four years of our marriage we went to enormous lengths to avoid me getting pregnant. We are both fit and healthy (in spite of my smoking) and didn't dream that there would be any problems when the time was right. I won't bore you with the horrors of the tests we both went through, but after eight years of trying we both reached the stage of believing it would never happen and were seriously considering adoption.

'Then the miracle happened. I won't attempt to explain the exhilaration. I couldn't wait for my husband to get home from work to share the good news. I'd been in the habit of carefully rationing out a packet of cigarettes a day, always leaving at least five for the morning. I went to light up and found I was down to my last two. It was only about five o'clock and I realized that I'd been chain-smoking since I'd got home. In the circumstances this was no great surprise to me. But the great shock was that it reminded me that I'd promised Eric and myself that I would give up if I was lucky enough to get pregnant.

In fact, one of the reasons that I'd looked forward to conceiving was to give up smoking! Far from looking forward to it, suddenly all my exhilaration was replaced by sheer panic.

'I didn't tell Eric. Although he's never been a smoker, he has always been considerate and never nagged me to give up, even though I know he hates smoking. I'm now in my fifth month, it's beginning to show and I still haven't told him. At first I made the excuse that it was too early and I didn't want to raise his hopes only to have them dashed. I now know that the true reason I haven't told him is that I cannot face the thought of attempting to stop.

'How can I expect him to understand, especially after all the trouble we went through? I feel so depressed and miserable. I couldn't feel worse if I had been unfaithful to him – and that's how I do feel, that I've been unfaithful to him. I'm not a stupid person in other ways, but I'm struggling to keep it down to two packs a day. I know that it would be better for me to tell him than wait for him to find out. And I know you believe that any smoker can find it easy to give up and that's what you'll advise me to do, but I still can't face the thought of even trying.

'They say: "Judge not lest ye be judged." I nearly lost my best friend because I harangued her for smoking five-a-day during pregnancy. Boy is she going to have a field day when she finds out about me! It's not as if I don't believe that smoking affects an unborn baby's health. I do. I know what it's doing to me and I keep having nightmares about giving birth to a deformed monster. Even that doesn't make me stop. I'm sure I'm a hopeless case and don't suppose you can help me.'

I didn't advise Jean to attempt to 'give up'. Instead I suggested that she should come along to the centre with her husband. I would explain to both of them the terrible power that nicotine addiction holds over its victims. She wouldn't then feel so guilty and self-despising and her husband would be better equipped to understand her predicament.

Jean was very well aware of the effect nicotine has. She thought, 'The power this evil holds over me is so great that I'll never be able to escape it, let alone find quitting easy.' The 'power' is in the panic feeling of believing that you cannot enjoy life or cope with life without a cigarette. That panic feeling is real. But once you understand that each cigarette, far from relieving the panic feeling, is actually the cause of it, that power not only ceases to exercise any control over you, but actually becomes the most powerful force to prevent you from craving another cigarette. Jean grasped this important point during our session.

Some people find it difficult to see this clearly while they are still in the misery of addiction. But you can see it if you are free of it. Both Jean and Eric were intelligent people. At the end of the session, he put his arms around her and said, 'I understand now. Don't even try to stop unless you want to.' Bear in mind that, at this stage, he still didn't know that she was pregnant. Her reply was: 'I've already smoked my last cigarette.' Then she told him about the baby. I've experienced hardship, setbacks and many sad moments during the twenty or so years I've fought a war against drug addiction. But the scene I was privileged to be a part of more than compensated me for those many difficult times. Ironically, the other witness to the joy was a large box of tissues.

Jean's was an extreme case, but only in degree; in substance it is all too common. It infuriates me that our society makes it so easy for young girls to get hooked; they are almost forced into the trap. We wait for them to become pregnant, then, at what is probably the most stressful period in their lives to date, and the time when they believe they most need their little 'friend', we subject them to massive pressure designed to shame them into giving up. Pregnancy has become a catalogue of tests, options, decisions, joy, excitement and fear. If they fail the quitting smoking test at this time, we treat them with contempt and berate them for their 'weakness'.

This attitude is understandable from the medical profession, even though it's not particularly helpful to either the mother or the unborn child. But non-smokers, ex-smokers, relatives and strangers feel justified and obliged to add their bit of abuse. Even the girl's smoking friends will join the witch-hunt with comments like, 'I just can't understand you smoking now that you're pregnant. I'd definitely stop if it were me.' Their attitude changes, however, when it is them; then they are able to see the other side very clearly. This inability to empathize is typical of human nature, unfortunately. When you've got a bad cold and are feeling very miserable with it, how many times has someone commented irritably, 'What are you making such a fuss about? You've only got a cold!' Usually the only time you will get sympathy is when someone else has a similar bug and knows from first-hand experience how bad it makes you feel.

Some girls are lucky: as nature alters their eating habits to benefit both mother and baby during pregnancy, they lose the desire to smoke. This is another example of the miraculous functioning of the human body.

Other girls make a conscious decision to stop, but fail. Even if the baby is born healthy, their failure, which was really no fault of their own, leaves them with a guilty conscience for the rest of their lives. It's hard to imagine what miseries they suffer if the baby is born with some defect.

Some women succeed in quitting smoking during their pregnancy, then after nine months of discomfort, fear, expectation and excitement, comes the most stressful period of their lives, the fear, pain, mental and physical exhaustion of the labour, culminating in the miracle of the birth. If all is well with both mother and child, the fear has gone, the pain and exhaustion are momentarily forgotten. The mother is instantaneously lifted from the lowest of lows to the highest of highs. These are the two extremes in a smoker's life, when the brain is triggered to shout:

I NEED A CIGARETTE!

Some women who stopped smoking for the major part of the pregnancy tell me that they lit up before the cord was cut or immediately after. Some resist the immediate impulse and are then caught out during the post-birth depressions. Regrettably very few stop permanently because of pregnancy. Like all reasons for stopping, once the reason no longer applies, neither does the desire not to smoke.

One woman who found she lost the desire to smoke during her first pregnancy, but got hooked again immediately after, told me she deliberately got pregnant again, not because she wanted another child, but to help her to stop. Initially it struck me as somewhat bizarre, but the more I thought about it the more sense it made. The problem was it didn't work.

Many pregnant girls either refuse to believe the adverse effects that smoking has on their unborn child, or justify them by saying: 'I think I would do the baby more harm by attempting to stop at this stage.' Some claim that their doctor actually forbade them to stop for this reason. I could write a separate book about the statements doctors have purportedly made about smoking. No doubt some of them are accurate reports of what doctors have said, but I think most of the attributed quotations have been taken out of context or embroidered. Another favourite defence of smokers is to re-use a justification put forward by another smoker on the basis that if it applies to that smoker it must apply to all.

At one of my seminars a young girl suffering from asthma declared that her doctor had told her that she had to smoke in order to relieve her asthma attacks. She made this statement in front of about thirty other smokers. I said: 'But smoking is a major cause of asthma. I find it difficult to believe that your doctor actually gave you this advice.' She confirmed that he had. I said: 'That's scandalous! Please give me his name and address and I'll pursue the matter.' She then began to backtrack: 'Well, he didn't actually say that, but I told him that when I had an asthma attack, a cigarette seemed to help me and he nodded.' Had I not pursued the point, thirty other smokers would have left that seminar with the impression that some doctors maintain that smoking relieves asthma.

Motivated by the best of intentions, many doctors advise pregnant mothers to try to cut down if they cannot stop completely. The advice sounds logical, but, as I have already explained, it is the worst of the three choices that the mother has. Instead of being subjected to the withdrawal from nicotine, whether it be mental or physical, for just a few days, she suffers the extra stress of this self-imposed restriction for the whole nine months and also guilt when she exceeds the intake limit on a bad day. But the really damaging aspect is that it ingrains into the mother's mind the illusion of just how precious each cigarette is. The waiting in anticipation of relieving that itch is present and growing. Once the cigarette is lit the relief is enormous and becomes a reward for having resisted. After the birth the mother is in the same position as a dieter who can no longer sustain the feeling of deprivation. The dieter goes on a binge; the smoker goes on an orgy of smoking.

Now, I don't intend to detail the ways in which smoking can affect, injure or even kill an unborn child, partly because enough has already been written about them, but mainly because the last thing a pregnant woman wants to read about is the damage she is causing her baby. She already knows about it, and it has not caused her to stop.

What all these well-intentioned people who criticize pregnant girls don't seem to realize is that the person who is most aware of the damage is the girl herself. She might not admit it to you, and she might try to justify her actions, but she already feels guilty about what she is doing. She is simply behaving as all smokers do throughout their lives. The more anxious, uptight and insecure other people make her feel, the greater is her need for the illusory crutch.

Apart from the pregnancy itself and the vilification that goes with it, pregnant girls are often hit by an additional shock at this time. Most smoking youngsters are convinced that they are in control and could stop if ever the need arose. Pregnancy is often the event that makes them realize they are just one among millions, another nicotine 'junkie'!

There is one aspect of the effect smoking has on a baby's health that I do feel bound to mention. I have read that babies whose mothers are addicted to heroin will themselves suffer withdrawal symptoms. This seems perfectly logical. After all, the same blood courses through the veins of both mother and foetus. It follows that the same principle should apply to nicotine addiction.

I know that when I tried to stop by using the 'willpower' method, I got very uptight because I wasn't allowed to have a cigarette. I also know that once I became aware that the empty feeling was being caused by the cigarette and would soon go, not having a cigarette didn't bother me in the slightest. Now, I have only known those two situations. One in which I believed the cigarette relieved the empty feeling and the other in which I knew it caused it. I do not know what it is like to suffer the physical discomfort of withdrawal from nicotine without relating it to cigarettes one way or the other. So how can I gauge what this is like?

There is one useful guide we can use. I have said that the physical discomfort from nicotine withdrawal is identical to a hunger for food. Babies are programmed to cry when they are hungry. A baby that is suffering the physical withdrawal effects from nicotine will feel permanently hungry and will keep crying. Feeding it won't satisfy that feeling. The tired and confused mother will tend to overfeed it and by doing so will simply exacerbate the problem.

Let's get back to the point. Be you pregnant or otherwise, I want you to stop smoking for the purely selfish reason that you will enjoy life so much more. I am not saying that there aren't genuine problems in life. If you have a genuine problem and you are able to do something about it, do it! If there is absolutely nothing that you can do about it, accept the fact – worrying about it won't help one bit. If you are a smoker, you do have a serious and genuine problem. Fortunately there is a simple and easy solution to it:

STOP SMOKING!

When you do you might well find – as did I and thousands of others – that those other apparently intractable problems suddenly evaporate. Either way, no matter what your problems or hang ups are, whether they be genuine or illusory, once you have escaped from the smoking trap, they won't feel nearly as bad as they do today.

Next we will address another illusion that is close to the hearts of millions of women:

THE MYTH THAT SMOKING HELPS
TO REDUCE WEIGHT

18 *The Myth That Smoking Helps To Reduce Weight*

I've lost count of the number of women who have told me that they deliberately took up smoking to lose weight. In fact, as I will shortly explain, smoking doesn't actually help you to lose weight. Like all the other illusions, it actually has the opposite effect. However, even if smoking did help to reduce weight, I don't believe any smoker deliberately chose to become a smoker for the rest of their life for that or any other reason. It is very important that you realize this. Other smokers are an important influence on getting us hooked in the first place, and in making us feel that we are missing out when we have managed to stop. It is important to understand that no smoker smokes because they choose to, or want to, that they are receiving no benefits from smoking, and all smokers wish they had never started.

What would you think if I used this same argument in relation to another damaging practice? For example, if I said, 'Not a single person, past or present, has decided to make a regular practice of placing their hand in boiling water in order to get the relief of removing it.' You might think this is so obvious as to be worthless as an argument. The real difference between the two is that with smoking we are fooled into believing that it gives us some genuine pleasure or crutch. I think we can agree that if we could see smoking as it really is – as 'devastation' – no one would choose to get hooked. But, as is so often pointed out, we are brainwashed into believing that we receive certain benefits from smoking. So why wouldn't someone be fooled into deliberately taking up smoking to obtain those benefits?

Even if we believe in the illusory benefits of smoking, we have no logical reason for becoming hooked deliberately. What are these illusory benefits? That smoking is pleasurable? The first cigarette tells us it's a pleasure we could well do without. We are told that it helps us to concentrate and to relax, and to relieve stress and boredom. But we also know that it is unhealthy, filthy and disgusting. Up to now we've been perfectly able to concentrate, relax, enjoy social occasions and even to cope with boredom and stress without breathing filthy fumes into our lungs. So why would we logically risk the downside for benefits that we don't actually need?

It just isn't logical. In fact, the only logical reason for deliberately becoming hooked would be to commit suicide. Even that wouldn't be logical, because if you genuinely wished to shorten your life, it is hard to imagine a more prolonged, painful, expensive and ineffective method of achieving this goal.

Nevertheless you might argue that an overweight adolescent anxious to attract a partner might believe that smoking helps to reduce weight and deliberately go through the learning process in order to do so. But let's credit our youngsters with a modicum of intelligence. Wouldn't a person of even limited intelligence know that the only sensible solution to losing weight would be to cut down on the quantity and type of food and drink they were consuming? The issue of body image projected by the media and the corresponding rise in eating disorders became such a hot issue in the 1990s that government intervention was sought to prevent the overuse of emaciated models, both male and female, in an attempt to curb the trend.

The advertising of cigarettes has changed radically, and the most powerful persuaders of the 'sexiness' or 'coolness' of smoking are not being peddled openly by the tobacco companies themselves. When youngsters see the likes of Kate Moss and other slim, attractive fashion/media stars puffing away, they want to buy into that image. What they are being sucked in by is free advertising for Big Tobacco. It's sad to think that these beautiful people are being used by the tobacco companies, and are not being paid a penny for it. In fact, they pay the tobacco companies to promote unknowingly an image that legally the tobacco could never achieve, and defend their 'use' of a product that will eventually kill them. All smokers are, in fact, working for the tobacco companies in this way, it's just that a few of them live in the media's eye and attract news coverage. Next time you are out, I'd like you to play a detection game. It's called spot the overweight smoker, and I guarantee you'll find it a real eye-opener.

Obviously a change of eating habits should be the first recourse to solving a weight problem. Surely no one would actually resort to deliberately getting hooked on the No. 1 killer disease in Western society and spending thousands during their lifetime just for the privilege, unless they had tried and failed by using more logical or conventional methods like dieting? You might think, 'perhaps they didn't believe they would get hooked and didn't work out what it would cost them'. I agree. In fact, a subtlety of the trap is that many teenagers dabble because they believe they won't get hooked. But that would hardly apply to someone who hasn't the self-discipline to control their food consumption. After all, we all know how addictive nicotine is and what massive willpower it takes to stop. This is why in the Sixties, when experimenting with 'soft' drugs was fashionable, many heavy smokers like myself were frightened to experiment, knowing that if we couldn't control our smoking, no way could we control what we believed to be harder drugs.

The fact that they didn't bother to work out what it costs them just proves my point. When we deliberately choose a specific course, usually we assess the pros and cons before making the decision. You don't just take up skiing; first you work out whether you can afford to, and, if you are my age, whether you want to risk breaking a leg, or worse. If it were a fact that one in three skiers died as a direct result of skiing, even reckless youngsters wouldn't take up the sport. Do you believe any smoker would deliberately take up smoking for any reason, let alone one as obtuse as losing weight, if they knew that their first cigarette would cost them a small fortune? In fact, if most of us had had to pay for our first cigarettes, we wouldn't have fallen into the trap.

Even when we have been hooked for many years and know that we are hooked, still we can't face working out the amount of money we have wasted and will waste in the future if we don't stop.

Ask a smoker how much they spend on smoking and they won't give you the true figure. Even when we are trying to 'give up', we bend the truth. We speak of saving so much money a week, when what we are actually doing is no longer squandering so much a week. You could argue that we sweeten the pill in exactly the same way when asked about our mortgage payments; we'll talk about only so much a month. Why we are so vague is for exactly the same reason; we don't wish to remind ourselves that we have a £100,000/$131,000 burden hanging round our necks. At least with our mortgage we faced up to the facts before we entered into the commitment. At times we might regard it as a burden, but the debt is for our most valuable possession: our home. It also happens to be an appreciating asset.

All smokers lie. They don't mean to. If they can find some seemingly logical explanation – such as 'I only took it up to lose weight' – they will cling to it. A cursory examination of such apparent 'logic' simply confirms that being a smoker is completely illogical. Smokers will spend hours trying to justify the reasons why they smoke. The fact that you won't find a single smoker in Western society who doesn't openly advise their offspring not to smoke is proof positive that no smoker continues to smoke because they choose to. Do you really believe that anyone would be so stupid as to pay tens of thousands to get hooked on a drug they didn't need until they got hooked, a drug that will shorten the life of one in three users and enslave them all for life? Even if you believed that smoking provided some genuine feeling of pleasure or support, every smoker knows that they didn't need it before they became hooked and that non-smokers aren't missing out. Every smoker instinctively knows that they have fallen into a trap. You don't need me to tell you that. What I want you to accept is that no smoker enjoys being a smoker, so don't envy them.

Many smokers will admit that they would love to be free. Others won't, and in order to save face they will bend the truth, just as you and I have done. But you will soon be free. Never forget that every smoker would love to leave the sinking ship. Don't envy them. Pity them.

Why do we believe that smoking helps to reduce weight? Whenever one of our friends brags that she hasn't smoked for six months, we congratulate her for looking so much healthier because of it. Secretly, though, we are thinking: 'That new wardrobe must have cost her a fortune!' It's true that most smokers who manage to stop using a 'willpower' method do put on weight. If your parents smoked, or an auntie or cousin, over the years you will have heard the immortal words, 'I tried to give up but I put on so much weight I started again.' Initially this has no real impact on you; only when we ourselves try to escape from the trap do we dredge it out of our consciousness as one of those incontrovertible statements about smoking. It has to be said that the weight gain is permanent for many ex-smokers. The obvious conclusion to draw from this is that as smokers put on weight when they stop, smoking must help to reduce weight. As with all other aspects of smoking, once you fully understand the nature of the trap, the opposite proves to be the true state of affairs. I can do no better than to illustrate my own case as an example.

I have already explained how the empty feeling for food and nicotine are identical and why a smoker is more likely to light a cigarette than eat a meal. Once we are hooked, eventually we tend to skip not only breakfast but also lunch. The evening meal then tends to take a more significant place in the smoker's mind; not surprisingly, as by this time of the day the body is genuinely hungry. When we've eaten this evening meal, we can be left with an empty feeling, even though what we've had was substantial. Naturally we believe that our hunger hasn't been satisfied, particularly as we've eaten nothing all day.

The true position is that during the day your body was demanding food but your brain interpreted the feeling as, 'I want a cigarette', so you smoked instead of eating. In the evening the body was craving nicotine, but the brain interpreted it as, 'You are hungry; eat more food.' In my own case, I didn't understand that my body was craving nicotine, and so I kept on eating. The empty feeling caused by the craving for nicotine is indistinguishable from hunger symptoms, and food won't satisfy a craving for nicotine any more successfully than nicotine will satisfy a hunger for food.

The result of this confusion is that we smoke all day in order to satisfy our craving for nicotine, but never satisfy our body's genuine hunger for food. Then we eat all evening to satisfy the craving for food, but don't manage to reach a state of feeling full, because our body continues to crave nicotine. Even though I didn't eat all day, I had still put on weight.

So why do smokers put on weight when they try to 'give up'? Because, although nicotine leaves the body very quickly, the 'little monster' does not die immediately and continues to crave nicotine for a short period. The natural tendency is to substitute food. I will explain later why substitutes make it more difficult to stop and are a major cause of hooking smokers again or ensuring that they continue to crave cigarettes even after years of abstinence. In such cases the 'little monster' has long been dead and the craving is purely mental.

We have now reached the most difficult part of the process: the stage at which, I believe, the smokers who fail when using Easyway founder. It is absolutely essential that you fully understand the point I am making in the next few paragraphs. Of the relatively small percentage of letters I receive from smokers who have so far failed to succeed, this extract from a letter sent to me by Barbara is most typical:

'Dear Allen,

'I know several people who have stopped smoking after reading your book. I agree it is a wonderful book and understand and agree with everything you say. I've read it several times, but unfortunately it doesn't work for me.

'I've tried several times but the longest I managed was three weeks. I'm a farmer's wife and we have four sons who all work on the farm. It is a very stressful life with long hours. Whenever I try to give up I can't stop thinking about smoking. I get very tearful and depressed. I know you're a very busy man, but I would appreciate it so much if you could help me.'

Before I can address the points raised in Barbara's letter, I need to give you some information that I've been keeping from you. I told you that there were only five instructions. This is true. But these were just instructions to follow while you were reading the book. They were designed to put you in the right frame of mind for when you smoke that final cigarette. There is another set of instructions designed to keep you in a happy frame of mind for the rest of your life. I have already addressed or hinted at some of them. Don't worry if you didn't notice them; they will all be itemized when the time is right.

Like selecting the correct direction in a maze, each of these instructions is important. One of them is not to even try to stop thinking about smoking once you have stopped. The reason I give this advice is because when we try to 'give up' using a 'willpower' method, we feel miserable because we are no longer allowed to smoke, but our mind is obsessed with the thought of smoking, and so we try not to think about it. But it's impossible not to think about something. If I say to you, 'Think of a huge pink elephant, covered with large black spots, trying to balance on a soccer ball', how could you possibly not think about it?

This brings me back to Barbara's letter. Quitting smoking is probably the most beneficial decision you will ever make. How could you possibly not think about it? Even if you tried not to, for a few days the 'little monster' would be reminding you that he hasn't been fed. You'd have well-wishers enquiring about your progress. You might even have smoking friends deliberately breathing cigarette smoke into your face and trying to convince you, and themselves, that you are missing out. It would be impossible not to think about smoking and if you tried you would only succeed in making yourself more miserable.

Why would you want not to think about it? It is not only the most beneficial decision you'll ever make, but the greatest achievement in your life. There's nothing bad happening; on the contrary, something marvellous is happening. After so many years of freedom, the subject of no longer smoking takes up about 90 percent of my waking and sleeping life. I still cannot get over the joy of being free.

Note that Barbara says: 'Whenever I try to give up, I can't stop thinking about smoking.' Obviously she still believes that she has 'given up' something, otherwise she wouldn't spend so much time thinking about smoking. She also explains that her life is stressful. I'm not disputing this, but if you had a stressful life, would you pay a fortune for something that greatly increased the stress?

Clearly, Barbara hasn't understood everything. Smokers who are having trouble stopping are not the only ones to misunderstand Easyway. Ironically, those who have succeeded in stopping often guide them into failure. If you'll recall, Debbie says: 'I don't even think about smoking any more.' Because smokers using a 'willpower' method feel deprived and miserable, they are naturally looking forward to a day when smoking no longer dominates their lives and they can stop thinking about it. Debbie's statement simply confuses them. It leads them to believe that the key to success is to stop thinking about smoking. The harder they try to stop thinking about it, the more obsessed and miserable they become.

The key is not whether or not you are thinking about smoking, but what you are thinking when you are thinking about it. If you are thinking, 'When will I stop thinking about it?' or 'When will I stop feeling miserable and deprived?', you are simply ensuring that the answer to both questions is, 'Never!' However, if you are thinking, 'Isn't it great! I'm already free!', you will be!

Is it really as simple as that? Is that really all you need to do for the rest of your life? Whenever you think about smoking, just think, 'Isn't it great! I'm already free!' No, it isn't. Also don't think that hoping that if you repeat it often enough will eventually make it come true. We know smoking is a fool's game. We never kid ourselves that it is chic or macho. You smoke because whenever you have previously tried to stop you couldn't concentrate, answer the phone, enjoy meals or cope with stress. You didn't understand why this was so, whether it was because of some flaw in your make-up, or there was some magic in smoking.

We didn't seem to understand why. We just knew that it was so. There is no way we could kid ourselves that being deprived of the 'crutch' was great or that we were free. Once you understand that the whole nicotine trap is a clever confidence trick, that you didn't smoke because of some flaw or weakness, that nicotine, far from helping concentration or relaxation, is actually the cause of your inability to concentrate or relax, then there will be no way that you can kid yourself that you need to smoke. When I think about smoking, I don't have to train myself to think, 'Isn't it great! I'm already free!' I knew I was, and I couldn't kid myself otherwise.

The reason smokers put on weight when they try to 'give up' is because for a few days the 'little monster' continues to create the empty, insecure feeling. The ex-smoker isn't allowed to scratch the 'itch', and since it's indistinguishable from normal hunger the obvious answer is to suck a candy or to chew gum. This inclination is reinforced by the fact that the ex-smoker has regarded a cigarette as a little reward to brighten an otherwise dull and stressful day and therefore needs a suitable substitute.

Obviously, ex-smokers are aware that chewing gum and sucking boiled sweets will make them put on weight. But they see it as a purely temporary measure and fully intend to stop doing it once they've kicked the 'habit'. The problem is that the sweet doesn't satisfy the craving for nicotine, and so they find themselves wanting another sweet and then another. Far from being a little reward, each sweet becomes stickier and more sickly. What's more, far from breaking the habit of a little reward, the sweets are actually perpetuating it. In no time at all, the ex-smoker is overweight, completely sick of sucking sweets and desperate for a cigarette. A valid excuse for having one has thus been created: 'I was not only killing myself being overweight but spending a fortune on new clothes. I thought I might just as well kill myself by smoking!'

Smokers who use 'willpower' methods do tend to put on weight for the reasons I've given. But be clear about this: they don't put on weight because they stopped, but because they fell into the trap in the first place. The nature of nicotine addiction is that it leaves you feeling permanently hungry and therefore more liable to become overweight. You might know smokers who are very slim, and have the shape of a supermodel. But, as Anita

Roddick, the founder of the Body Shop chain, once pointed out, there are only seven super models in the world; the rest of us are normal.

It is important to realize that most substitutes cause you to be overweight and miserable, and also actually make it harder for you to stop. I emphasize that there is no need to gain weight even for a short period when using Easyway.

Try to imagine the 'little monster' as a live tapeworm inside your body which feeds on nicotine. How long do you have to starve it before it dies? It is possible to do medical tests to ascertain how long it takes for all the nicotine to leave your body. However it is impossible to know when the 'little monster' ceases to crave nicotine. Why? Because the actual physical feeling is almost imperceptible and is indistinguishable from an empty, insecure feeling caused by a hunger for food and certain other aggravations that we will continue to live with. Therefore the estimates I give you are based on my own experiences when attempting to stop and on the observations and comments of thousands of other smokers. But please:

DON'T PANIC!

Forewarned is to be forearmed. Let me explain what you can expect so you will have nothing to fear. The moment you cut off the supply of nicotine, the craving gradually builds up and reaches a peak after about five to seven days. From this time onwards the ex-smoker gradually feels less tense and more relaxed. The body detoxes and returns to a state of homeostasis, or balance. After about three weeks of abstinence, the ex-smoker senses that the 'little monster' has died. You reach a state that formerly you couldn't visualize without smoking. Suddenly you realize that, not only haven't you smoked during this time, but the thought didn't even occur to you. You realize that you can enjoy life and cope with what it throws at you without being dependent on nicotine. You feel completely free.

This is a very pleasant feeling for any smoker, no matter what method of trying to stop they are using. It also happens to be a dangerous moment, one that has destroyed many otherwise successful attempts to stop. Because you feel free, you want to light a cigarette just to prove it. And it does just that! After three weeks of abstinence the cigarette tastes weird and foul. You get no feeling of pleasure or that nicotine is a crutch and are left wondering how you could have harboured those illusions. However, you've put nicotine into your system again, and the moment it starts to leave you, you've created a new 'little monster'. The probability is that you won't scratch the 'itch' immediately, but a few days or weeks later, when you might be tempted again, you think: 'I smoked a cigarette two weeks ago and didn't get hooked, so where's the harm?' You've landed in the same trap that you were in the first time round, and before you know it you're smoking as heavily as you were before.

It is important not to confuse this three-week period with the extended craving endured by smokers who try to 'give up' using the 'willpower' method. These smokers are not even aware of the 'little monster'. Long after it has died, whenever they suffer an empty, insecure feeling, whether it be caused by a hunger for food, normal stress or anxiety, joy, or whatever, their brains will still be saying: 'That means you want a cigarette – you still haven't kicked it!'

A moment ago I stated that when you cut off the supply of nicotine, the craving gradually builds up and reaches a peak after about a week. You might construe that you'll suffer severe withdrawal symptoms at this time and you'll have to endure a period of resisting the craving. Not so! Remember, the actual physical sensation is so slight that we are not even aware of its existence. This is why casual smokers can go a whole week apparently without experiencing undue aggravation. Also remember: that empty feeling accompanies you throughout your smoking life without you being aware of it, and it gets no worse when you stop.

When finally I stopped I couldn't understand why I didn't crave cigarettes or suffer withdrawal symptoms. I was immediately over the moon, and have been ever since. I've been referring to the cravings of the 'little monster'. In fact, the body cannot crave nicotine any more than it can crave food. All the body can do is send a signal to the brain, such as 'I'm hungry, I need to eat', or 'I want or need a cigarette.' The former is a safety device, like a fire alarm, to ensure that you survive and lead a long and happy life. But the latter is a cruel, subtle confidence trick. It is telling you that you want or need a powerful poison that will gradually destroy you mentally and physically and will provide you with absolutely no pleasure or crutch whatsoever.

Be aware that, particularly during the first few days while the 'little monster' still lives, you might have the feeling of, 'I want or need a cigarette.' Now we have reached the nub of what I consider to be the most important and crucial difference between Easyway and 'willpower' methods.

On a 'willpower' method the ex-smoker rationalizes the many powerful reasons why being a smoker is stupid. Yet, sometimes within just a few minutes of deciding you will never smoke another cigarette, part of the brain is saying, 'You want or need a cigarette.' This is very confusing. We don't understand that it is just the death throes of the 'little monster'. You assume that you want or need a cigarette because they provide you with some pleasure or crutch, or because you haven't yet broken the habit. The reason doesn't really matter. The fact is you want a cigarette but won't allow yourself to have one. This makes you feel deprived and miserable. Meanwhile, the 'little monster' hasn't been partially satisfied, and so the desire or need is gradually increasing. This makes you feel more deprived and miserable, which in turn creates distress.

Identify a key time when you need a cigarette. That's right – when you are under stress. It's a cause and effect situation: the greater the stress, the greater the need. The longer that need cannot be satisfied, the greater the stress. No wonder smokers 'giving up' with 'willpower' methods get so uptight and find it so difficult.

With Easyway you can expect to have the feeling of, 'I want or need a cigarette'. Accept this and when it occurs it won't faze you. You understand that it is just the death throes of the 'little monster'. You know that feeling is a cruel confidence trick, and you know it has been brought on by the previous cigarette. Because you know smoking provides neither pleasure nor a crutch, instead of craving a cigarette and feeling deprived and miserable because you can't have one, your attitude is the complete opposite. You say to yourself, 'Now I understand how this clever confidence trick works. No way am I going to be conned into breathing any more of this poison into my lungs. Isn't it marvellous? I'm free!' You get the opportunity to reinforce your understanding of the true situation every time you experience the physical effect of nicotine leaving your body.

You could argue that no matter what prompts the feeling of, 'I want or need a cigarette', technically you are still actually craving a cigarette. Not really: a verb with 'ing' on the end, such as breathing, eating or sleeping, implies an ongoing situation. A craving isn't an instantaneous feeling but a prolonged desire that isn't satisfied. Have you noticed how, when you buy a new car, the switch that operates the windshield wipers is always where the one to activate the indicators or horn was on your old car? It's typical Murphy's law. For a few days, whenever you want to indicate, you activate the windshield wipers or horn instead. Once I hit what I thought was the horn when a driver cut in front of me and simply sprinkled my windshield. Apart from feeling slightly stupid, no great damage was done. In fact, I would have completely forgotten the incident by now if Joyce didn't say 'Give him a squirt, Allen!' whenever another car cuts in front of us.

Accept that any changes in life, even ones for the better, such as a better car, job or home, take time to adjust to. When you hit the windshield wipers instead of the indicator, do you get all uptight about it? Do you insist on deliberately repeating the practice? Of course not; you just accept that it takes time to adjust, and get on with your life. Also remember that any minor inconveniences you go through when quitting are caused because you fell into the trap in the first place; they are not caused because you're trying to stop.

So, accept that in the early days of stopping smoking your brain will probably shout, 'I want or need a cigarette'. Realize that you are at liberty to make a choice. You can say to yourself, 'I'd love a cigarette now. How long will the craving last? Will I ever be free?' If you take this route, you will actually be choosing to crave; this would be unbelievably stupid of you. While you choose to act in this way you will never be free.

I have told you that no smoker chooses to continue being a smoker, and that smokers have fallen into a trap that they don't know how to escape from. However, be clear: there is a means of escape. Easyway gives any smoker a key to that prison. It gives you the choice to leave it immediately, easily and permanently. If and when you have that moment of 'I want or need a cigarette', instead of getting into a panic and bemoaning the fact that you can't have one, just stop and say to yourself: 'I understand this. It's simply the death throes of the "little monster". Isn't it marvellous? I'm already free!'

AND YOU WILL BE

But how will you know that you are not kidding yourself, that you are really free? You can't kid yourself that you are not dependent upon nicotine. Nobody is ever dependent upon nicotine, not even smokers. They were simply fooled into believing that they were. On the 'willpower' method, smokers put out what they hope will be their last cigarette and then spend the next few days saying: 'I'd love a cigarette, but I mustn't have one!' Some of them spend the rest of their lives never having a cigarette, but at odd times saying, 'I'd love a cigarette.' Pause for a moment. Just think of the stupidity of that situation: to say I want to be a non-smoker then spend the rest of your life periodically saying, 'I'd love a cigarette.'

Can you think of a worse case of muddled thinking?

What's the real difference between a smoker and a non-smoker? Non-smokers have no need or desire to smoke. Regardless of the method they are using, what are smokers really trying to achieve when they attempt to stop? Is it to go through life craving a cigarette at odd times and feeling miserable because they won't allow themselves to have one? Of course not! They cling to the forlorn hope that if they can abstain for long enough, they will wake up one morning with the feeling of:

ISN'T IT GREAT? ISN'T IT MARVELLOUS? I'M FREE! I'M A NON-SMOKER!

The one thing you can be certain of is that they won't. For the reasons I've already given, they conspire against themselves and ensure that they never will achieve that marvellous state. You don't need to wait to become a non-smoker. In fact, it is essential that you don't wait to become a non-smoker. If you put out what you hope will be your final cigarette, believing that cigarettes provide some form of support or pleasure, how can you possibly prove otherwise?

Doesn't it make more sense to remove all the mystery, confusion and doubt first? If you do this before you put out that final cigarette, you know there is nothing to give up, that smoking doesn't assist concentration and relaxation, or relieve boredom and stress, but is a major cause of boredom and stress and actually impedes concentration and relaxation.

Doesn't it make more sense to start off with awareness of the beautiful truth? That you are giving up nothing, that far from being deprived of some pleasure or crutch, you are simply being cured of Western society's No.1 killer disease and a lifetime of misery, poverty and slavery? Doesn't it make more sense to start off with the feeling of:

ISN'T IT GREAT? ISN'T IT MARVELLOUS? I'M FREE! I'M A NON-SMOKER!

That's what I did. That's what Debbie did, and that's what the hundreds of thousands of other ex-smokers who have succeeded with Easyway did. All you need to do is to follow the instructions for it to happen to you. If you start off with that happy feeling, you don't have to wait for something to happen:

YOU ARE ALREADY A HAPPY NON-SMOKER

– and can get on with the rest of your life rejoicing in that fact. If you wait to become a non-smoker, whether it be for five days, three weeks or longer, you will simply be waiting to achieve a state that you are already in. In effect, you will be waiting for nothing to happen.

Just as non-smokers and smokers have good days and bad days, so do ex-smokers. On a 'willpower' method, the ex-smoker tends to blame everything that goes wrong on the fact that they no longer smoke. On Easyway, expect things to go wrong, but be aware that the moment you put out that final cigarette, not only will the nicotine start to leave your body, but so will all the other bad effects. If you have heard reports that it takes between seven and ten years for all the effects to leave your body, ignore them: they have been put about by medical experts, who are trying to persuade you to stop now. Such scare tactics don't work; all they achieve is to frighten the life out of us, which makes us more likely to reach for another cigarette. Sure, scaring us reinforces our intention to stop, but tomorrow not today – and we all know that tomorrow never comes.

The effects of smoking never leave the body completely while there are smokers around; even non-smokers have traces of it, just as we all breathe in the other poisons with which we pollute the planet. However, the system that created us has made us incredibly strong. I don't know how I avoided lung cancer or the other killer diseases, given how much I smoked. But the fact that I did proves my point. I don't worry about inhaling the relatively small quantities I'm compelled to consume from smokers.

Be assured, though, that the bulk of the gunge leaves your body within a few days of quitting. Don't wait for it to happen! Just be aware that the moment you put out that final cigarette, you will quickly become stronger both physically and mentally.

When you have a bad day, accept it. Just say to yourself: 'OK, I'm having one of those days, but because I am physically and mentally stronger, I'm better off than I was when I was smoking.' You will soon discover, as I did, that the bad days will occur less frequently and the good days will multiply. When you are physically and mentally low, molehills appear to be mountains. When you feel physically and mentally strong, what you once viewed as major problems tend to become minor challenges that you enjoy accepting and overcoming.

If I appear to be repeating the point, I make no apologies for doing so: it is absolutely essential that you understand it. The 'little monster' is real, but it never craves. Like the rest of the brainwashing, it might be the catalyst to making you crave a cigarette, but you have the choice of whether you do or don't. At some time you must have turned on a tap and put your hand under scalding hot water. Did you leave it there while you decided whether or not to remove it? Of course you didn't. You have exactly the same choice if you catch yourself thinking, 'I need a cigarette.' Is it sensible to ponder the fact that you can't have one? If you do, what you are actually pondering is: 'Would I like to become addicted to "devastation"?'

During the few days after you put out your final cigarette, if and when you get the empty feeling, how will you know whether it's the death throes of the 'little monster' or a genuine hunger for food? You won't know, any more than you know while you remain a smoker. The point is that you don't need to know. During that period, you are going to eat sensible meals and you are not going to pick at snacks between meals. In other words, if you get the empty feeling you will assume that it is the death throes. They are hardly noticeable anyway, and far from letting them trouble you, you are going to rejoice in them.

Perhaps you are already a compulsive eater and cannot resist picking at food between meals. If so it's probably because you are addicted to nicotine. I have already explained why this leaves you feeling permanently hungry and reinforces my point that smoking doesn't help you to reduce weight. If you already have a weight problem, you have nothing to lose. On the contrary, you will probably find that solving your smoking problem will also solve your weight problem and most of your other problems, as it did those of hundreds and thousands of other smokers who have followed the instructions of Easyway.

Bear in mind that even if you fill yourself with sweets or cookies you will still feel hungry. You will also deny yourself one of the truly great ongoing pleasures of life. When you fill yourself with sweets, not only do you get fat and miserable and completely sick of them, you also ruin a most precious commodity: a healthy appetite. It's not just a quaint custom that in cultures where food is appreciated, prior to a meal you are wished a 'good appetite' rather than 'good food'. Even good food isn't enjoyable unless you are hungry. We tend to regard hunger as unpleasant. It isn't. On the contrary, it is essential to the genuine pleasure of enjoying a good meal. Eat regular, sensible meals and you won't be aware of being hungry between them.

Even if you experience hunger for those few days when you first stop smoking, that's no great ordeal. Hunger is a precious commodity, and the longer it lasts the more enjoyable that meal will be when it comes.

Smoking actually increases the feeling of hunger, but at the same time ruins your senses of taste and smell. One of the great advantages of quitting is to enjoy the return of both senses. And you can do so the moment you put out the last cigarette. However, if you use sweets or cookies as substitutes, you'll not only deprive yourself of those pleasures, but you'll also get fat and miserable. Several other bad things will also happen. In due course I'll be addressing the importance of breaking down associations and removing the void; substitutes perpetuate both. They also ensure that you never know when you are free. Even if substitutes worked, you would then be faced with the problem of 'giving up' the substitute.

It's time to take stock of our progress. In Chapter 7 I asked you to complete a questionnaire composed of common illusions that are generally accepted as facts. Let's ask ourselves:

HOW MANY MYTHS HAVE WE EXPLODED?

19 *How Many Myths Have We Exploded?*

Consider each of the original questions put to you in the questionnaire on page 68. Take your time, and when you are ready, make a note of your responses. When you have done this, compare them with the responses you gave before. Are they different?

Now read the explanations that follow each of the questions below. Where necessary, refer back to relevant chapters to ensure you understand the points made.

1. Do smokers smoke because they choose to?

   We have firmly established (Chapter 7) that smokers no more choose to smoke than they choose to speak their native tongue. Did the American tourist who bought London Bridge choose to buy it? No one forced him to make that purchase, so you could argue that he made a choice. But he was the victim of a confidence trick. He didn't choose to be conned. Does a mouse choose to eat the cheese in a trap, or an insect choose to eat the nectar of a pitcher plant? No doubt they would have chosen not to if they had known the full facts. They were conned!

2. Do people smoke out of habit?

   No, they smoke because they fell for the most subtle and ingenious trap that man and nature have combined to set for them: NICOTINE ADDICTION (Chapter 5).

3. Are long-term smokers more hooked than teenagers? (Chapter 5)

The 'experts' are confused about the question of when a 'dabbling' youngster actually becomes hooked. When does the insect become hooked? That's obvious: when it first gets the scent of the nectar, it has no choice other than to follow its natural instincts. Youngsters get hooked the moment they decide to light that first experimental cigarette. So why don't all youngsters who try an experimental cigarette get hooked? For the same reason that some fish or mice who take the bait don't get trapped – they were lucky!

As to whether long-term smokers are more hooked than teenagers, you could equally ask –

4. Are heavy smokers more hooked than casual smokers? (Chapter 9)

Who would you envy the most: someone trapped in quicksand up to their ankles or someone who is up to their neck in it? They are both in the same trap. Who has the best chance of escape? Is it the ones who don't realize they are trapped and believe that they smoke because they enjoy smoking and choose to smoke? If you realize that you are in a trap and want to escape, at least you have a chance. But if you have no desire to escape, your chances are zero!

5. Do youngsters start smoking to feel adult, 'cool' or rebellious?

There is no doubt that youngsters do like to feel adult and 'cool'. Aren't childhood and adolescence just training grounds for adulthood? A rebellious spirit is surely a quality rather than an evil, provided it has good intentions and receives good guidance.

I have four children. I'm happy to say that all four had a rebellious streak. I tried to impress upon them the stupidity of being a smoker. I also taught them the Green Cross Code. Two of them started smoking. After I had impressed upon them the importance of the Green Cross Code, not one of them found it necessary to play 'chicken' when crossing the road. In fact, I don't know of a single case of a child rebelling against the Green Cross Code. So why do our naturally rebellious children rebel against not smoking but don't rebel against the Green Cross Code? Doesn't it suggest that they take up smoking for another reason?

Ironically, teenagers don't see grown ups smoking as chic or 'cool'. Rather they regard them as idiots for having become addicted! They have no way of understanding the trap, nor can they imagine ever getting that old. Do you remember Christine's daughter, Sarah, who was crying because she thought Mommy would die? In all probability she's now hooked on cigarettes herself. I remember watching my father coughing his lungs up. There was nothing chic or 'cool' about his watering, bloodshot eyes, his nicotine-stained fingers and teeth or his bad breath. But did this prevent me from falling into the trap? Of course not, and it doesn't prevent hundreds of thousands of youngsters from falling into the trap today. Shy youngsters admire their rebellious peers. Smoking is still adopted as a badge of independence, a form of cutting loose from parents, an integral part of the rite of passage into adulthood. Aside from these valid reasons, though, they smoke for exactly the same reason that you and I did. They were conned!

6. Are smokers stupid?

If they are, Bertrand Russell, Freud, Einstein and even Sherlock Holmes were stupid. Yes, I know Sherlock Holmes is fictional, but isn't this all part of the brainwashing and confusion? Holmes talks about a 'three-pipe problem'; the great man couldn't activate his powers of deduction without smoking. I should imagine only a few youngsters nowadays read about Sherlock Holmes. His modern-day equivalent would probably be Mel Gibson's character in the *Lethal Weapon* movies. Is it surprising that we believe we can't concentrate without a cigarette? Is a mouse stupid for nibbling at the cheese? We would say so, because we know that cheese is bait. Is an insect stupid for alighting on a pitcher plant and sampling the nectar? Again, we can understand how that particular trap works and wouldn't fall into it.

But the nicotine trap is something else. It's ingenious, designed by human beings to attract human beings. Just a few generations ago it had trapped 80 percent of the adult, male population. It still traps over 30 percent of our youngsters, and now more girls than boys. It is responsible for the early demise of more people than any other single disease, starvation and the combined war casualties of the history of our planet. Nicotine addiction currently claims over five million victims every year. The World Health Organisation has estimated that the figure will rise to ten million by the second decade of this century.

Do you think mice would nibble at the cheese if they understood exactly how the trap worked? Telling our children that smoking is expensive and bad for their health clearly doesn't prevent them from falling into the trap. They are no more stupid than you or I are, and the trap is identical to the one you and I fell into. What will prevent them from falling into the trap is an explanation of exactly how the trap works. Simply telling them that smoking ruins their health won't dissuade them.

Many years ago I was the only advocate for Easyway. Now there are thousands who can vouch for my claims. They know that Easyway works. When you have satisfied yourself of this fact, I would be grateful if you would do more than just write to thank me. Please write to the media, your doctor, your member of Parliament and ask them why they persist in perpetuating the illusions that enable this particular blight on our planet to flourish. Encourage them to come out of the

Dark Ages and into the 21st century. It is a sad fact that only when smokers contract lung cancer do they realize the true nature of the trap. Then they will ruminate on their stupidity and blame themselves. But this is unfair. They were simply victims of a clever trap that could have been avoided if they had understood it.

What greater gift can we pass on to our youngsters than the information that will give them at least a fighting chance of avoiding the nicotine trap? Even rebellious youngsters are open to approaches that don't involve trying to scare them away from cigarettes, as our therapists who go into schools to give talks about smoking know from the feedback they've received.

7. Do smokers enjoy the taste of some cigarettes? (Chapter 5)

8. Do some cigarettes (e.g. after a meal) taste better than others?

If smokers ever actually ate a cigarette, we'd know the answer to both questions. If you have ever smoked a roll-up or made up a butt from the ashtray, you will know what tobacco tastes like and will therefore know exactly what I mean.

Some smokers claim to smoke because they enjoy the smell of tobacco, yet all smokers when walking into a smoky atmosphere will cough and comment on how unpleasant it is. The difference is that a smoker acclimatizes far more quickly than a non-smoker and very soon fails to notice the atmosphere.

We need to address this question of tobacco fumes smelling pleasant. Non-smokers will tell you that the smell is actually foul, particularly when they are enjoying a meal. However, at other times even certain non-smokers will appear to enjoy the smell of tobacco. They too are beginning to feel the effects of addiction and be attracted to it. You don't have to smoke yourself to create the 'little monster'. The worst aspect of passive smoking is that those carcinogenic fumes include nicotine and this component can actually create the 'little monster' in non-smokers. The effect can be particularly potent in ex-smokers at two important times, both of which you need to be aware of.

One of those times is the first few days after you have put out your final cigarette. The 'little monster' is starving and crying out to be fed. To the ex-smoker who is unaware of the nature of the trap they've just escaped from, the smell of a burning cigarette can be as tempting as the scent of nectar is to an insect. It is that band of ex-smokers who you see trying to waft the smoke from a cigarette past their noses. The smell triggers a learned response that associates lighting up with feeling comfortable. Now, if you have recently stopped smoking it can be disconcerting to find yourself suddenly, out of nowhere, recognizing that old I-Want-A-Cigarette signal. Ex-smokers who are in the position of knowing what this is all about don't get into a flap. They take note of what's happening and use the moment to be grateful that they no longer have to light up. They know the feeling will soon pass.

It is also important to realize that tobacco and cigarette or cigar fumes only appear to be pleasant when you are not actually smoking. Some pipe-smokers will sniff their tobacco pouches prior to lighting up, just as you might sniff a delicious stew before satisfying your hunger. Neither the smell nor taste of tobacco is pleasant once the 'little monster' has been satisfied.

But shouldn't you avoid passive smoking if it addicts you again? No! Get it clear in your mind: it is not the 'little monster' that addicts you. What addicts you is the 'big monster': the belief that some pleasure or support can be got from feeding the 'little monster'. The piece of cheese tricks the mouse into falling into the trap. But if the mouse could understand the trap, it would see that piece of cheese as it really is: a piece of bait that would break its back, not as food that would satisfy its hunger. Incredibly, with the smoking trap, the bait isn't even food, but the No. 1 killer poison in Western society. Once you understand the trap completely, no way are you going to be tempted to feed the 'little monster'.

The other important time you need to be aware of is social occasions, particularly over Christmas and New Year when parties are rife and you've been subjected to an inordinate amount of passive smoking. You might have noticed that the people who are most aggressive about your smoking are not those who have never smoked, but the self-righteous ex-smokers (HTTs, or Holier Than Thous). Having spent the bulk of their lives defending their freedom to smoke if they want to, they stop for a week and belligerently defend their right to breathe air unpolluted by filthy and inconsiderate smokers. It's not so much that they are inconsiderate or even lacking in compassion themselves. It's more that the passive smoking has recreated the 'little monster'. Even if the tobacco doesn't smell pleasant, they can hear that little siren voice saying, 'You really would like a cigarette.' Ex-smokers feel vulnerable at such times. They know that they are better off than the smokers, but the smokersseem happy and cheerful and are allowed to smoke. Their antagonism towards smokers is a defensive reaction. By attacking and humiliating smokers, they are reinforcing to themselves the correctness of their decision.

So is the answer to avoid other smokers? This sounds logical, and is what the 'experts' advise, but in reality it's just as unfeasible as trying not to think about smoking. Just consider for a moment what it might involve. It would mean you couldn't go to any social function, wedding, funeral, party, bar or restaurant where there might be smokers. If you have friends who smoke, you would need either to drop them or become an HTT and insist that they didn't smoke in your presence. If there are smokers at your place of work you would need to change your job. You couldn't go to your golf, tennis or bridge club because smokers also go there. And if your partner happens to be a smoker, and the inconsiderate so-and-so refuses to stop and insists on smoking in your presence, you would have to seek a new partner. The only choice left to you would be to join an order of nuns or live in some other type of commune where smoking was banned. And imagine what else you would have to forgo to fit in to either.

There is absolutely no need for you to avoid smokers and smoking situations. You're not trying to give up living! In fact you haven't even 'given up' smoking. There's nothing to give up.

The moment you put out that final cigarette you will have solved the problem. You will have ceased to poison your body and will rapidly become physically and mentally stronger. You can start enjoying your life immediately, provided of course that you don't start moping for support or pleasure that never actually existed. Nothing could illustrate this better than what I refer to as the 'dinner party' incident.

I had met Margaret once before, but she had got embarrassed smoking in front of me. People know what I do for my living and assume that I'm bound to be the worst HTT they are ever likely to meet. They assume that I'll lecture them about the evils of smoking. It so happened that on this second occasion, she was the only smoker present. I don't think she was worried about offending anyone by smoking, but just felt self-conscious because she was the only smoker. Anyway the meal was over and she had the 'smoker's twitch'.

Everyone else was chatting away but Margaret sat fiddling with her lighter and cigarettes. I can't bear to see smokers in this state, so I said, 'Margaret, the meal is over, no one will complain, have a cigarette if you need one.' She replied, 'I don't need one, but I would like one.'

I should have shut up really, but her response was like waving a red rag under my nose. I just couldn't resist commenting, 'If you don't need one, leave it. There's no point in choking yourself if you don't need to.'

She was about to light up. Instead she just said: 'Fine, I'll leave it.'

I continued conversing with Shelagh, the girl next to me, who I hadn't met before, but my attention remained with Margaret. I wanted to see how she would cope with the situation. Of course, before long the twitching became unbearable.

No doubt your sympathies will be with Margaret. As smokers, I'm sure you've suffered many similar situations in your life, as I did. But get it clearly into your mind: I wasn't the real villain of the piece. That filthy weed was the real villain. Non-smokers don't have this problem of being miserable when they are not allowed to smoke. At one point Margaret got up to go to the powder room. She picked up her lighter and cigarettes, glanced across at me and immediately sat down again. I can only assume that she thought that I would have made some facetious remark. I was now beginning to feel petty. Far from easing the situation, I had made it worse. I was trying to think of a way to get over the impasse, when Shelagh suddenly said: 'I'd murder for a cigarette now.'

I was truly surprised, because I knew she was a non-smoker. In fact, I was convinced that she had never been a smoker. She was one of these delicate types, like fine porcelain. She had a beautiful complexion. But I think what actually fooled me was that she was a church minister's wife. Why a clergyman's wife shouldn't smoke, I don't know. Most of them probably do. But you get preconceived ideas about people.

I said, 'I'm sorry, I didn't realize that you were a smoker. If you are not smoking because of me, don't think you will offend me. I was the world's worst.' She said, 'No way! I haven't smoked for eight years, and I will never smoke again. But I used to love a cigarette after a meal and I would really enjoy one now.' Meanwhile Margaret, who believed I was now genuinely occupied with the minster's wife, had lit up and was taking a sneaky drag.

The incident amply illustrates the total futility of being a smoker. On the one hand there was Margaret, looking decidedly guilty and uncomfortable, snatching sneaky puffs on her cigarette, hoping that no one had noticed that she had lit up and wishing she were free, like everyone else in the room. On the other hand there was Shelagh, who hadn't had a cigarette for eight years, actually moping for something that she herself hoped she would never have!

It was a ridiculous situation. It's stupid to envy someone else, even if you believe her life is better than yours. Here you had a situation where the women envied each other, yet each had the choice to be smoker or non-smoker. The annoying aspect for me was that I had spent half an hour before the meal chatting to Margaret, gently telling her how nice it was to be free and persuading her that she could do it. I had a rope around her waist and was gradually easing her out of the pit. Margaret was one of those smokers that had never managed to survive a whole day without a cigarette. Can you imagine the effect it had on her when she heard that Shelagh was still craving after eight years?

A national newspaper recently devoted a whole article to a woman who had decided to start smoking again after eight years of abstinence. In the article the woman went into elaborate detail about the misery of those years and how she had gained pounds in weight. She described how wonderful she felt when she made the positive decision to smoke again. Most of all she eulogized about how gorgeous that first cigarette tasted.

Now, I have every sympathy with that woman. I have referred to my miseries when attempting to stop by use of the 'willpower' method. I am also very aware that I greatly exaggerated the trauma. I have no doubt that she wasn't a happy non-smoker, but let's examine her statements more closely. If she thought smoking was so great, why did she stop in the first place? If her eight years were so bad, why didn't she give up her attempt much earlier? The fact that she didn't would imply that she hated being a smoker. I cannot believe that it gave her any pleasure when she finally had to admit to herself that her eight years of 'penance' had been a complete and utter waste of time!

I can remember an enormous feeling of relief when I finally allowed myself to give up the struggle during those failed attempts to stop using the 'willpower' method. But I cannot once remember thinking, 'Great! I'm a smoker again. Doesn't this cigarette taste absolutely gorgeous?' On the contrary, that feeling of relief was always tempered by a feeling of failure and foreboding, and the first few cigarettes tasted weird.

Diarrhoea is unpleasant, but to someone who has been constipated for eight years it must seem like utter bliss. I've no doubt that if you've waited eight years for a cigarette, the relief would be immense, but not the taste. As I've said before, all drug addicts are liars. They have to be. Shelagh's remark at the dinner party was quite harmless, even so its effect on Margaret was devastating and completely negated my earlier chat with her. Can you imagine the effect that newspaper article had on someone who had recently 'given up', who was going through the miseries of the 'willpower' method or a smoker contemplating an attempt to stop?

You've no doubt witnessed or been involved in situations similar to the dinner party incident and can empathize with the woman in the newspaper article. Even so, don't avoid the presence of other smokers. On the contrary, other smokers can be the most potent reminders of just how wonderful it is not to be one for the rest of your life! Scratch the outer surface, look behind the self-deception and see all smokers, casual or otherwise, as they really are: miserable drug-addicts. Once you get a real look at them, your only feelings for them will be of pity.

If the thought of a party without smoking still frightens you, make a point of attending one as soon as possible after you've smoked your final cigarette. But don't go with a feeling of apprehension. Nothing bad will happen. You will have escaped from a life sentence of imprisonment for a crime you didn't commit. On the contrary, something exciting and marvellous is happening.

You are about to achieve what every smoker on the planet aspires to: FREEDOM. It is your opportunity to prove that you don't have to wait to become a happy non-smoker. You can enjoy life, including meals and other social events, immediately. You will be the prima donna, the centre of attention. Those smokers will be expecting you to be complaining and miserable. Even when you are the only non-smoker present, every one of those smokers will be envying you. Some of them might be too scared to admit it. Some might blow smoke in your face or deliberately offer you a cigarette when they think you are off-guard. Don't despise them; pity them. The fear that nicotine addiction engenders can cause otherwise pleasant and compassionate people to act like barbarians. You might find yourself on such a high that you forget you have stopped, and find yourself reaching for one of those cigarettes. Before you can take it, the offerer exclaims, 'I thought you had "given up"!' This is followed by smug laughter from the smokers. You stand there, arm stuck out in space, embarrassed and deflated, thinking: 'I thought I'd "given up" too!'

This is one of those significant situations we've already discussed that causes doubt to creep in. You'll ask yourself: 'Am

I really free, or am I just kidding myself?' Don't worry, all you did was to hit the horn instead of the indicator. Just think, the mere fact that you had forgotten is a marvellous sign. What better proof could you have that not only can you enjoy life immediately, but your thoughts don't need to be obsessed by the fact that you no longer smoke.

There are various ways you can react to that proffered cigarette. You could accept it, then screw it up with some comment like: 'I had no intention of smoking it. I just wanted to remove a nail from your coffin.' However that's not my style. Those smokers will probably have sensed that you had genuinely forgotten. They would also have sensed that you were on a genuine high about being free. You can do no better than to be completely honest with something like: 'I can't believe it. On previous attempts I was so miserable and was obsessed with the thought that I wasn't allowed to smoke. If anyone had told me that after just two days I could forget that I no longer smoked and would actually get immense pleasure from refusing a cigarette, I wouldn't have believed them!'

You might think that such a reply is a bit pointed. In fact you'll be doing those smokers a favour. Be aware that a constant battle of bluff rages between smokers and ex-smokers who have 'given up' with a 'willpower' method. The ex-smokers will keep going on about how much healthier they feel and how much money they have saved and what a filthy, disgusting habit smoking is anyway. The smokers will enthuse about the pleasure they receive, that the money is well spent and that they could step under a truck tomorrow. When you stop with Easyway you don't have to bluff. You have a 'Royal Straight Flush' and you know the smokers don't even have a pair of twos. Even with smokers who genuinely love you and want you to succeed, part of them will want you to fail. The reason is that you will have joined the millions who have escaped from the sinking ship, reinforcing every smoker's fear that eventually they will be the only smoker left on it.

It's those complaining ex-smokers like Shelagh, and the woman in the newspaper article, who make even the thought of 'giving up' so terrifying. So, don't avoid smokers. When they see that you can enjoy life immediately, and genuinely not miss smoking, they will think you are Superwoman. You'll then have the additional pleasure of inspiring your family and friends to stop. But, more important, you'll actually feel like Superwoman. Cast away any lingering doubts you might have and look forward to what so many Easyway advocates describe as the greatest achievement of their life. Like anyone who is released from a jail, the elation of being free will never go.

Another common theme in the letters I receive is the belief that it is impossible to stop if your partner smokes. Don't make the mistake of trying to persuade them to stop at the same time. If you do, you'll either lose them, or even if they go through the motions, they'll secretly want to undermine your success. Even if you succeed, you'll probably turn them into the unhappiest individual on the planet: a secret smoker! Just follow the above principles. When they realize that you are genuinely free, they'll join you of their own accord.

We have now exploded illusions 1 to 8 inclusive.

Myths 9 to 12 inclusive are best dealt with collectively.

9. Does smoking help to relieve boredom?

10. Does smoking help you to concentrate?

11. Does smoking help you to relax?

12. Does smoking help to relieve stress?

I've already stated that relaxing and stressful situations and boredom and concentration are complete opposites. Ask a smoker how the same cigarette manages to achieve the complete opposite to the one smoked an hour earlier; even the 'experts' are at a loss to explain this phenomenon. In fact, there is a very simple explanation. When nicotine leaves a smoker's body it causes them to feel stressed and tense. If a smoker is in a genuinely stressful situation, such as a car accident, they will assume that the stress is due entirely to the accident. When you light up and actually feel less distressed than a moment before, the brain is fooled into believing that the cigarette has partially relieved the genuine stress. What you don't realize is that even while smoking the cigarette, you are actually more distressed than if you were a non-smoker. This is because the cigarette only partially relieves the withdrawal syndrome. In a relaxing situation, smokers cannot feel completely relaxed while they are in the grip of the 'itch'. This explains why even casual smokers tend to chain-smoke at parties. Don't just take my word for it; observe for yourself.

Boredom and concentration require a little more explanation. It's almost impossible to convince a person who has a job that entails long periods of boredom (a night-shift worker, for example) that a cigarette doesn't relieve boredom. It's rather similar to someone believing that chewing gum helps you to relax. One of the symptoms of stress is to grind one's jaw. All the chewing gum does is to give you another reason for grinding your jaw. It might well save some wear and tear on your teeth, but relieve stress it does not. If chewing gum genuinely relieved stress, the sufferer would have no need to go on chewing it. Again, don't take my word for it; next time you see someone chewing gum, ask yourself whether they look relaxed or under stress. The true situation becomes so obvious when you remove the brainwashing.

The only reason that we believe that smoking relieves boredom is because we tend to light up when we are bored. But boredom is a mind problem. When it occurs it's telling us that we have nothing interesting to occupy our minds. It's easy to see how doing a crossword puzzle, reading an interesting book or taking up some absorbing pastime could genuinely help to occupy our minds. But smoking a cigarette isn't a particularly mind-expanding activity. Even the lighting up process becomes automatic after a while. I agree that those first experimental cigarettes for a group of children might have been instigated out of boredom and actually succeeded in relieving it for a few minutes. Once we are hooked, though, smoking becomes subconscious. When you light up because you are bored, do you suddenly think, 'My word this is interesting. I breathe these cancerous fumes into my lungs and then breathe them out again. What jolly fun this is!' We don't go through this mental process even when we smoke the so-called 'special' cigarettes, such as the one after a meal! Just as chewing gum doesn't relieve stress, but simply serves to emphasize your unrelaxed state, so smoking, far from relieving that boredom, simply emphasizes the fact that you are bored.

So why do smokers smoke when they are bored? Partly because they have been brainwashed to believe that smoking relieves boredom. Mainly though it's because while you have something to occupy your mind that doesn't involve stress or concentration, you won't be aware of that 'itch'. However, if you are genuinely bored, you have nothing to take your mind off the 'itch' and you will keep scratching it.

Just think of my situation: chain-smoking cigarette after cigarette, day after day for over thirty years. Have you the imagination to visualize anything more boring, more disgusting or more stupid?

Nicotine addiction is a major cause of boredom for several valid reasons. Because we believe it relieves boredom, it is the easy option and prevents us from seeking genuine solutions to boredom. Because it makes us feel lethargic and strains our finances, we don't have the energy or money to take up genuinely interesting pursuits. But most important of all, because we feel increasingly uncomfortable in situations in which we cannot smoke, we avoid those situations. Was it just coincidence that I stopped playing soccer, rugby, cricket and tennis years before my non-smoking peers? Was it just coincidence that my passion became golf, which enabled me to exercise and smoke at the same time?

I've said that doing a crossword puzzle provides a genuine antidote to boredom. True, and many smokers wouldn't even contemplate doing a crossword puzzle without a cigarette. I was one of them. To concentrate effectively, it is necessary to remove all distractions. Smokers have a permanent distraction: the 'itch'. You don't need to be aware of it. This is why most smokers will light up before making a phone call. It's always more difficult to communicate over the phone, so first you remove all possible distractions. If it's a stressful call, you have an additional reason for lighting up. If it's a chat with a friend, you still need to feel completely relaxed. And if she happens to be a bore, it's essential that you have an adequate supply of cigarettes. Again, lighting up only partially relieves the 'itch', so you are less able to concentrate than if you were a non-smoker.

A very famous and otherwise competent Oxford professor has stated on national TV: 'Smoking definitely helps the concentration.' We've all been brainwashed to believe this to be true. If it is true, why don't we make it compulsory for train drivers, pilots, surgeons, or for that matter, those who do any job that involves a high level of concentration, to smoke during working hours? Why are they positively forbidden to smoke during working hours? It's because we instinctively know that it's only people who have fallen into the trap who cannot relax, relieve boredom or stress, or concentrate without nicotine.

During my many attempts to 'give up', I found it impossible to concentrate without a cigarette. This was because I believed that smoking helped me to concentrate. Whenever I had a mental block, I would sit there, not trying to solve it, but thinking that a cigarette would solve the problem and bemoaning the fact that I wasn't allowed to have one. No mystery as to why I couldn't concentrate!

Is it only smokers and ex-smokers who experience mental blocks? If it is, smoking would appear to cause them rather than relieve them. Of course everyone has mental blocks from time to time. What do non-smokers do when they get one? They do exactly what smokers used to do before they became hooked: they try to find a solution. Because the 'itch' is only partially satisfied when we light up, smoking actually impedes concentration. The degeneration that nicotine sets in motion affects every organ, including the brain. After I stopped smoking with Easyway, I continued to get mental blocks, but because I knew that smoking ruins concentration, I didn't waste time moping for a cigarette. I put my mind to searching for a true solution to the block. I had a mental block while trying to write this chapter. When I was a smoker I would have lit yet another cigarette. I know that having a cigarette is not the solution, but a distraction, and so now I look at the situation logically. After a few moments reflection, the cause of the block and the remedy for it became apparent to me. I'd been concentrating solidly for five hours – my brain needed a rest. And so I stopped working. It's amazing how seemingly insurmountable problems miraculously disappear after a good night's sleep!

We have already exploded myths 1–12 inclusive, let's now deal with two of the most enduring fantasies in the smoker's imagination.

13. Do smokers enjoy smoking?

Even when you understand the nature of the trap and how the illusion works, it is very difficult to accept that you have never actually enjoyed smoking. It is even more difficult to comprehend that there's not a single smoker, past or present, who has enjoyed smoking a single cigarette, cigar or pipe. You have to remove the illusions and all the brainwashing to come face to face with the true situation: that nicotine addiction is no more or less than DEVASTATION, as defined at the beginning of Chapter 6. Re-read that definition and you'll find it difficult to comprehend how anyone could be deluded into believing that they did enjoy smoking.

Ask a smoker why they smoke and the answer is usually something like: 'Obviously because I enjoy smoking.' Ask them what it is they actually enjoy about breathing filthy cancerous fumes into their lungs and they immediately become less articulate. We have already exploded all the more detailed excuses that smokers come up with and proved that they are just illusions. I know many women that admit to wearing tight shoes. I've yet to meet one who admitted to enjoying the experience. In a restaurant they are usually discreetly removed at the same time as another aggravation – the need to satisfy the 'itch'. Smoking is equivalent to wearing tight shoes; neither experience is enjoyable.

However, there is one reason occasionally offered by the more discerning smokers as their reason for smoking, which I have not yet addressed: the ritual. Consider this extract from a letter:

'I'm a qualified psychiatrist and a very heavy smoker. I know I'm not a fool and have deduced that I must get some pleasure from smoking otherwise I and all the other millions of smokers wouldn't smoke. I've analysed all the usual reasons that smokers give but none of them seem to make sense. For some time I believed the only explanation was that I had an addictive personality, but my professional training enabled me to see that that didn't make sense either. I've come to the conclusion that

it is just the ritual that is enjoyable: the beautiful packaging, removing the cellophane and the gold leaf paper, offering the packet to a friend, extracting the perfectly rolled and packed cigarette, the lighting, those first few inhalations and even more satisfying exhalations, provided of course you aren't sitting next to a non-smoker! I associate this ritual with some of the most pleasant moments of my life and, frankly, I just can't visualize life without it.'

This letter raises two other important points, but let's address the ritual first. If it were the ritual that was so pleasurable, it would be possible to continue with the ritual but not actually light the cigarette. Smokers have tried doing this but found that it only works for a short period. David Bryant, for many years the top exponent of lawn bowls, would actually keep an empty pipe between his lips during indoor tournaments when he wasn't allowed to smoke. It's easy to understand why it doesn't work if you appreciate the ritual of eating.

Call me a snob, but I love the ritual of a meal at a restaurant with nice decor, pleasant atmosphere and a picturesque view. If it's with waiter service in the company of good friends, so much the better. The clean linen, cut-glass, silver and attractive china all add to the pleasure of the ritual. Now imagine the smell of your favourite food has been permeating the atmosphere and you are ravenous. Finally the food is served. You sit politely waiting for your companions to be served. You are about to taste the first mouthful when the waiter taps you on the shoulder and says, 'So sorry, but you're only paying for the ritual not the food.' Would you enjoy the ritual if you weren't allowed to eat? Of course not. You'd be absolutely livid. The whole object of the ritual of a meal is to enhance your pleasure at satisfying your hunger. If you are unable to do that, the ritual would be pointless, unpleasant and exceedingly frustrating.

With smoking, the attractive packaging, gold lighters, silver cigarette cases and cut-glass ashtrays serve the opposite purpose:

to delude you into believing that there is something pleasant or sociable in breathing filthy cancerous fumes into your lungs. But just as the ritual of a meal would be pointless without being allowed to eat, so the ritual of smoking would be pointless without being allowed to scratch that 'itch'.

Another way of highlighting this phenomenon is when you try to smoke those herbal cigarettes that you can buy from drug stores. I needn't say any more if you have smoked them. If you haven't, go and try them; you'll see exactly what I mean.

14. Do some people have addictive personalities?

I particularly like this claim because it is impossible to prove that something doesn't exist. What you can do is to weigh all the evidence, use your intelligence and decide which is the more likely possibility.

Many smokers come to the conclusion that they have an addictive personality. Why? Usually because it's the only rational explanation. But even if there were such a thing as an addictive personality, still it doesn't actually make sense. If I had a gregarious personality, it would mean that I like mixing with other people. I would set out to do that and actually enjoy doing it. Consequently, an addictive personality would mean that I wanted to become addicted, not just to nicotine, but to heroin and any other addictive substance. I've yet to meet anyone who deliberately set out to become addicted to a drug.

The whole subject is irrelevant. Let me put this argument to you in the most compelling form I know. If I were to give you a million pounds to fund research into why more Egyptians than Ukrainians drown in the Nile, and to establish whether the Egyptians have an addictive personality trait which causes them to drown in the Nile, it wouldn't take you long to assess the situation and come up with a conclusion. Ukrainians don't drown in the Nile because they don't live near it. The Egyptians don't have an addiction to drowning; they drown only when bathing in or boating on the Nile. You aren't addicted to heroin because you don't use it. You can't be addicted to anything unless you use it first. Amazingly this revelation hits thousands of smokers who believed they had addictive personalities until they tried Easyway.

It's not your personality that addicts you, but an addictive drug. What also addicts you is the belief that you get pleasure and/or support from the drug, and that you cannot enjoy life or cope with stress without that drug. In other words, you are dependent on that drug to help you survive the stresses and strains of life. Sure you're physically addicted to the drug, but you are also addicted to the illusion that without cigarettes you are not whole. Once this illusion is exploded, so is the addiction.

We have now exploded myths 1–14 inclusive. Before we explode the remaining six, we need to address the other matter raised by the letter earlier on: 'I associate this ritual with some of the most pleasant moments of my life, and frankly I just cannot visualize life without it.' We need to discuss the importance of:

REMOVING THE ASSOCIATIONS

20 *Removing The Associations*

Easyway will work for any smoker. But, no matter how hard my colleagues and I try to ensure that it does work for every smoker who attends one of our centres, a small percentage of smokers don't succeed. Although they might refer to themselves as failures, we never do. We know that each one of them can find it easy to stop. Our motto is the same as that of the Canadian Mounties: 'We Always Get Our Man' – or Woman! In all cases where success is proving difficult, we attempt to analyse the reasons. All the instructions are important, but I would ask you to pay particular attention to the following points, which appear to be the main reasons for failure:

THE BELIEF THAT YOU ARE DIFFERENT AND THAT EASYWAY WON'T WORK FOR YOU

This is negative thinking, pure and simple, and will defeat you before you start. Should you try but not succeed at your first attempt with Easyway, it means you haven't understood or followed one or more of the instructions. This is easily remedied. Except in one important respect, you are no different from any of the other 40 percent of the world's population who fell into the trap and are trying to escape. You are in possession of the true facts, not mumbo-jumbo or guesswork. You are now equipped with a clarity of thought that previously eluded you.

STARTING IN A DEPRESSED AND FEARFUL FRAME OF MIND, BELIEVING THAT STOPPING IS GOING TO BE VERY DIFFICULT

What's there to be depressed about? You are choosing to be free. It's not every day you get to feel like Nelson Mandela on the brink of release after years of imprisonment. Start off in a happy, confident frame of mind, and see stopping as an exciting challenge. You have absolutely nothing to lose and so much to gain.

FAILURE TO UNDERSTAND THAT THE ONLY REASON ANY SMOKER CONTINUES TO SMOKE IS TO FEED THE 'LITTLE MONSTER'

That 'little monster' is the purely physiological addiction in your body, and the notion that smoking gives you either pleasure or support is simply an illusion created by the 'little monster'. The monster creates the disharmony and discomfort you feel inside. Your brain, seeking to remove that feeling, mistakenly believes that a cigarette will fix the imbalance. You understand this chain of deception now, and realize that when you light up, each cigarette, far from removing the empty, insecure feeling, actually perpetuates it. The permanent cure is to get rid of the monster altogether.

NOT UNDERSTANDING THE FACT THAT THE 'LITTLE MONSTER' WILL SURVIVE FOR A FEW DAYS AFTER YOU PUT OUT YOUR FINAL CIGARETTE

When you've put out that final cigarette, you may well find yourself suddenly wanting a cigarette. Remember, this is not you consciously wanting a cigarette. It's just the 'little monster' in its death throes. This is the time to rejoice and to confirm your decision.

FAILURE TO RECOGNIZE AND THEN BREAK DOWN THE ASSOCIATIONS IN YOUR MIND

This brings me back to the windshield wipers analogy. All of us have traits that stem from old patterns of behaviour. Some people twiddle their hair when nervous as a form of comfort; something they did as a child. Smokers tend to stress the negative aspects of not being able to smoke. We can't imagine being able to use the phone or attempting to solve a difficult problem without a cigarette. This is because we associate being miserable with not having cigarettes. The fear of being miserable forever in ALL situations is enough to put anyone off even attempting to stop smoking.

If at the outset of your attempt to stop smoking you find it difficult to visualize a meal without a cigarette, what is likely to happen? I'll tell you. You'll stop for, say, five days. Then you'll go out for a meal with friends. After the meal they'll light up, you'll get the whiff of nicotine and the not-quite-dead 'little monster' will cry out to be fed. What will you do? You'll either use willpower to resist the temptation to light up, or you'll light a cigarette. After five days of abstinence, it will taste weird, but the relief of scratching that 'itch' will partially satisfy the 'little monster', extend its life and ingrain in your mind the illusion that no one can enjoy a meal without a cigarette.

While you remain fearful of these associations, you'll have to use willpower to resist lighting up. And it's not only the 'little monster' that triggers, 'I want or need a cigarette!' Any of the associations we've discussed will do it. This is why Shelagh could still 'murder for a cigarette', even after eight years of abstinence, and why smokers who use willpower to 'give up' never feel completely free.

It is essential to break as many of the associations as you can think of before you put out your final cigarette. This will involve some imagination on your part and might even take courage. But the rewards are great. Remind yourself of these. Tell yourself that is what you are going to do.

First, get it clearly into your mind that all those situations you associate with smoking were, and will be again, intrinsically pleasant. You have adequate proof of this already without needing to refer to anything that you have read in these pages.

You know that non-smokers have no need or desire to smoke at such times. You also know that you didn't either before you fell into the trap.

Remember that your smoking actually impeded your pleasure at such times, because of the learned pattern of behaviour that only addicts suffer from. In other words, when a smoker cannot smoke, any situation deteriorates rapidly and the moment is no longer unconditionally enjoyable. It is only the cigarette that creates this misery. If you approach those situations as a non-smoker with the frame of mind of the smoker, you won't enjoy them. If you're thinking, 'I don't think I'll be able to enjoy this situation without smoking', you are deliberately ruining your chances of success.

In the last chapter I recommended that you attend a party as soon as possible after you have stopped. Do this, but use it as a proving ground. Look for the associations, think about them, use them to change the thought patterns in your conscious and subconscious mind. If you do this you can re-write the programming. Prove to yourself that you don't have to wait to become a non-smoker or even endure a period of misery. Just as you will enjoy the bad effects of smoking leaving your body, you will enjoy removing the poison from your brain by removing the associations.

There are literally dozens of associations. Let's address a few of the more typical ones.

You meet a crowd of smokers at a wedding or on vacation. They're all laughing, happy and obviously having a good time. The cigarettes are passed around and it's easy to think, 'This isn't fair; these people are obviously having a good time. They can smoke and I can't.' Of course they are having a good time, and the reason is not because they are smokers. They're on vacation. Although they won't all admit it, every one of those smokers will be envying you. If you start craving a cigarette in such circumstances, you'll be craving for a situation that never existed. You'll be on a loser to nothing: either you'll make yourself miserable because you can't have one, or you'll make yourself even more miserable because you do.

Imagine that those smokers had a disability other than being victims of the smoking trap. Let's say they had all lost a limb. They could still be having a great time on vacation, but would you start to feel that you were missing out because you were lucky enough not to have that disability?

Closely associated with vacations, airport lounges are also traps for ex-smokers, particularly if your flight has been delayed. How they manage it I don't know, but wherever you sit, you seem to be surrounded by packets of duty-frees. You are bored and frustrated and you can hear smokers gloating over the money they have saved. It's easy to sit there thinking, 'I used to save a fortune on duty-frees. I'll just buy the one packet.' Don't! Instead, remind yourself that far from making any saving, on average those smokers are going to spend tens of thousands in their lifetime just for the privilege of enslaving themselves and destroying their health.

Take a closer look at those smokers around you, particularly those on the same delayed flight. See if they look happy and cheerful.

Expect to find yourself in situations where old associations present themselves. These are your Pavlovian bells. Because women are more in touch with their emotions and recognize them immediately, they tend to come to the surface readily, especially upsetting ones. When we experience disharmony we will try to remedy the situation by seeking out an action, thought or solution. Be prepared for them.

If and when those bells do start ringing, reinforce your decision by understanding that your first reaction – 'I want a cigarette' – is nothing more than a conditioned reflex, a shadow memory that is responding to discomfort.

If a trauma befalls you during the first few weeks of stopping smoking, this feeling may be quite intense. But, remember, there are two forces at work here, not just one:

You may still be in the late stages of purging the nicotine from your body and thus it is physically in a state of turmoil.

You are suffering from the mental aggravation of the traumatic event.

Your brain won't automatically split the difference and say to you: 'Half of this is physical because of nicotine withdrawal and the other half is because you're emotionally upset'.

YOU WILL JUST FEEL STRESSED!

Having learned, like Pavlov's dogs, to respond to the bell, and believing the cigarette will relieve the feeling, you will get the trigger to light up. But you know that cigarette will only ever offer a temporary relief and, worse still, that it will start the whole process off again.

Don't panic when this trigger presents itself. Use its occasional appearances to remind yourself of the reality. Never question your decision to stop. Remind yourself how lucky you are to be a non-smoker.

Other classic situations are life's mini-dramas. Someone crashes into your car. Naturally you are not too pleased about the situation. You start to think, 'At times like this I would have had my little crutch.' Think back to the time when you were a smoker and had mini-dramas, or major ones for that matter. No doubt you did light a cigarette, probably several, but can you ever remember thinking, 'Isn't life wonderful? I've smashed up my lovely car, but who cares? I've got this gorgeous cigarette to smoke.' Again, by even contemplating having a cigarette at such times, you would be simply torturing yourself.

A less common, but often more critical situation can be the reunion with that special friend who was your smoking partner for many years. Perhaps you noted that Emma Freud was greatly influenced by the friend who had started smoking at the same time. However, the influence can be equally strong in reverse. You've been in the habit of reminiscing about past experiences and getting up to date with current progress, all with a glass of wine and a cigarette. How could it possibly be the same without a cigarette? You worry that your friendship might be blighted in some way.

Do you remember Emma's remark?: 'They had left the club and I hadn't.' Won't that get-together make your friend feel uncomfortable and make you feel like a traitor? Prepare yourself for such situations in advance. Remind yourself that you haven't left a social club, more like a leper colony. Never forget that no matter how your friend might try to convince you otherwise, she would love to be free, like you.

Note also that it took seven of Emma's friends to escape before Emma herself would admit that she hated being a smoker. Just think of the satisfaction the original friend got from helping so many friends, including Emma, to escape. You'll soon be enjoying the same pleasure.

If smoking could do everything we claim it does, up until your final cigarette would you not agree that you would have been –

**TOTALLY Stress-free
ALWAYS Relaxed
NEVER Bored and
ABLE to concentrate at all times?**

Who was it who created the expectation that somehow we were missing something to make us complete?

The sixth and greatest reason for lack of initial success with Easyway is:

THE 'VOID'

21 *The 'Void'*

What is 'the void'? It is the belief that by whichever means we evolved on this planet somehow we are incomplete. Whether you believe we were created by a god or evolution, or a combination of both, doesn't affect the situation one bit. We accept that the more advanced species such as gorillas, tigers and elephants are physically incredibly strong and can survive in the wild without the benefit of artificial clothing or shelters, without hospitals, doctors, drugs, medicines, injections or vaccinations.

You could argue that all these species are in danger of extinction. That is only because an even stronger species has virtually monopolized the planet and has not only destroyed their habitat and polluted the rivers, land and very air that they breathe, but has butchered these magnificent creatures for purely commercial and aesthetic reasons to obtain ivory, furs and hides.

We regard gorillas, elephants and tigers as incredibly strong animals physically, and yet we are constructed of exactly the same skin and bone. Indeed, we are informed that our DNA is roughly 96 percent the same as that of the chimpanzee. It is also indisputable that for a much greater length of time than we have been on this planet, homo erectus survived without fire, let alone hospitals, doctors, drugs and the comforts and safety nets we take for granted.

Why, when a baby giraffe can walk within a few hours of birth, does it take a human baby a year? Why in Western society is a completely natural function like childbirth treated as though it's a disease? An aboriginal mother can give birth with only another woman in attendance, and twenty minutes later be up and about.

I'm not suggesting for one moment that we should revert to a primitive way of life. Nor am I disputing that modern medicine has helped reduce the mortality rate of both mothers and babies. I'm simply pointing out that we seem to have evolved to the point where we believe not only that a baby is physically fragile, but that we adults are both fragile and incomplete.

How often have you heard that old phrase: 'Schooldays are the happiest days of your life'. The stupid thing is that we believe it. Birth is the most stressful experience that any creature goes through. The fact that Mother Nature is kind and allows us to be unaware of, or soon forget, this experience doesn't alter the situation. Childhood and adolescence are also stressful times, during which we are learning to cope with life, to mature and to become independent. Once we've achieved independence and maturity, our lives should be all honey and roses, but they're not. The excuses we give are the mortgage, the taxing job and the worry and responsibility of feeding, clothing, educating and generally raising a family. We enter into all these responsibilities voluntarily, so why do they become stressful responsibilities rather than pleasures?

It is because from birth we are brainwashed and conditioned to believe that we are in need of some miraculous product or gadget to be better, to become whole. In truth the human body and mind combined make up the strongest and most sophisticated survival machine on the planet. Compared to elephants and tigers, we believe that we are far superior mentally and far inferior physically. In truth it's the complete reverse. If schooldays are the happiest days of our lives, why is the incidence of adolescent suicides in Western society increasing every year? Why are we the only species on the planet that has learned to cry, let alone commit suicide?

Our so-called intelligence is being used to destroy us. Adolescence is a genuinely stressful time, but like all other creatures on the planet, nature has equipped us to cope with it. I truly believe that the best survival device we have at our disposal is our conscious mind. In other words, we have the power to reason.

In Chapter 18 we addressed how the ingenuity of the nicotine trap causes us to light up whenever we suffer an empty, insecure feeling, regardless of whether the feeling is due entirely to nicotine withdrawal, as when relaxing after a meal, or caused by normal stress. We have got into the habit of lighting up whenever the empty, insecure feeling occurs. We are fooled into believing that the cigarette is relieving that feeling. But now you understand the nature of the confidence trick. Just as you quickly adjust to the changes in your new car, you are quickly going to reverse the habit of seeing a cigarette as relieving the empty feeling, and feeling deprived because you can't have one. You are going to see a cigarette as the cause of the problem and rejoice in the fact that you have no need to continue the chain of persecution, because the problem is already solved.

All the time we remain in ignorance of the true facts about the nature of the confidence trick, there are those who will use every trick in the book to continue to exploit our situation. Consider the following.

The tobacco companies have for decades been using psychoanalytical tactics in their marketing campaigns. Information gathered by government and industry has revealed that people generally desire and acquire products to boost themselves. The average person wants to be someone and material products are seen as a means of giving them a higher status in society. Seizing on this trend, the tobacco companies set about gathering their own information to enable them to target specific social groups with their products.

They hired eminent psychoanalysts to work closely with marketing departments to come up with the right logo and image to fit the wants and desires of these groups. Colours and ideas associated with young adulthood, success and social integration were used to capture different markets. This work is still going on, obviously successfully, as the tobacco companies are still succeeding in trapping generations of smokers.

Documents subsequently leaked and used in legal process against the tobacco companies reveal just how cynical are the marketing ploys they use. The smoker is described as 'illogical and stupid' about their addiction. In short: they have no idea we are pushing a highly addictive drug, and even those who reach that conclusion cannot break free.

You would have hoped that after the discovery of such information there would have been worldwide governmental intervention to prevent the marketing of cigarettes. But sadly not. The release of these documents during the Minnesota trials against Philip Morris Inc. et al in 1998 has had no effect on the activities of the tobacco industry, and has not galvanised governments to oppose them. It's still business as usual for the tobacco companies.

Some of the information they rely on comes directly from you. Sales, for example, are regularly monitored by means of information they receive from shopping surveys. You may well have completed one of these surveys yourself. Although they don't come from the tobacco companies directly, they get sold on to them. In future make sure you tick the data protection box to prevent the forwarding of the information you give.

In the 1960s the ratio of male to female smokers stood at 60:40. Thereafter the trend was downwards; the number of male smokers declined by over 50 percent, to 27 percent, while the number of female smokers fell to 30 percent, a 10 percent drop. The tobacco companies concluded from these statistics that men seemed more successful at getting out of the game than women, so much so that by 1998 only 28 percent of men were smoking; at the same time the percentage of women still smoking had only gone down to 27 percent. By the 1990s women were now seen as the plug that would stop the bottom falling out of the market for cigarettes in the Western world. Women, the tobacco companies' research revealed, seem to be less influenced by anti-smoking campaigns, mainly because these were perceived to be geared towards male smokers and did not apply to women. The issues raised in the campaigns had very little resonance for women, which could account for why women seem to find it more difficult to stop.

The rate of female smokers now equals that of men. More alarmingly, among teenagers the rate for girls is rising fast, and in some countries they are actually out-smoking the boys. The main driving force behind this rise is the successful marketing strategy of Big Tobacco. From the 1960s onwards they cashed in on the profound change that occurred with women's liberation and the corresponding increase in the economic independence of women. The industry quite clearly regards women as a market to be conquered and a large portion of the annual advertising and marketing budget is aimed in their direction. Documents subpoenaed from the companies revealed systematic analysis by segmentation of the market to better respond to the emerging 'wants and needs' of modern women. An enormous amount of research has gone into targeting this market.

Most alarming of all are the notes about under-age female smokers, and the development of a lifestyle approach to market products aimed at these youngsters. They seek to identify women's views and desires, and also to exploit current trends and predict future trends. They talk of image-enhancement brands that stand for contemporary femininity. The key to this piece is in the tobacco industry's stated aim: to 'counteract the effects of everyday life'. 'Women,' they state, 'look for ways to withdraw and regain... not only will this product provide an escape' [for example, when the children are playing up and screaming blue murder], 'but it will also serve as a reward' [the 'I'll just finish off the housework/weekly reports/thesis and then I'll deserve a cigarette break for having been so good']. Sounds all so familiar, doesn't it?

If you smoke Marlboro Lights, they have caught you well and properly. In fact, any brand which flies under the banner of 'lights' is a con. This product was aimed at the health conscious and designed to represent a major step in reducing harm, thus providing the smoker with an apparently legitimate reason not to stop. By their own admission the tobacco companies state these cigarettes 'are nothing more than a scam'. You just take in deeper breaths to get out the level of nicotine your body 'needs' to feel balanced. If you doubt this, think back to when you last smoked an ultra light. (Yep, you covered up the holes with tape, didn't you?)

Last but not least the tobacco companies have developed products specifically aimed at women on low incomes. What better than a flash of gold on a packet to give the illusion of grandeur and wealth?

Take a look at the chart opposite. I've no doubt you can spot yourself in one of the categories that Big Tobacco has identified, all the better to understand women smokers by. (If you are interested in finding out more about the world of the tobacco industry, look on the Internet under Big Tobacco.)

I could go on and on about the tactics devised to get you into the smoking trap. Just acknowledge that you could not possibly have imagined anything quite so elaborate or sinister when you lit that first cigarette.

You can now use this information to reinforce the new perception you have of cigarettes, to keep from getting back into that prison which that chart illustrates so clearly. They say hindsight is a wonderful place to be. In this particular instance you have lived through the reality of being a smoker. You didn't like it, that's why you read this book: to escape. Being a smoker can never get better, only worse. If you hate the position you're in now, you'll always hate it. If you could go back in time to that very first cigarette, what advice would you give yourself?

You will soon be in the unique position when you put out that final cigarette, when you end the nightmare and walk free. You will take yourself back to a time when you could enjoy life as if you had never lit that first cigarette. With all that you know now, you can give yourself the best advice. At last you can make an informed choice.

YOU CAN STAY IN THE TRAP FOR THE REST OF YOUR LIFE, IGNORING THE REALITY 99 PERCENT OF THE TIME, KNOWING HOW MISERABLE YOU ARE AND WILL ALWAYS BE

or

YOU CAN SET YOURSELF FREE AND CELEBRATE THE JOY OF ESCAPE

How Big Tobacco sees you

Information taken from 'A Structural/Psychological Segmentation of the Adult Female Market'

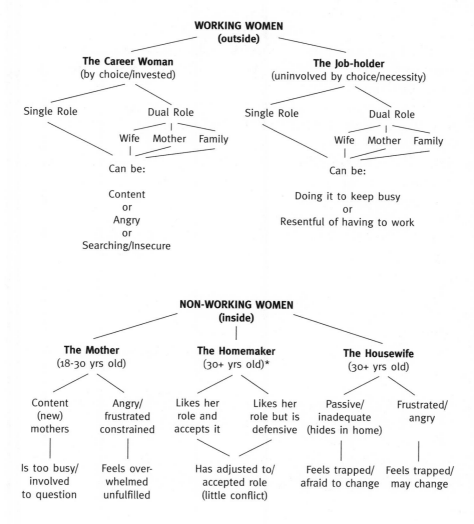

* The ages are given as reference points only. There are fewer and fewer women, aged 18-30, who do not have children and are not in paid employment.

The void never existed before that first cigarette. Since that day you have been trying to fill a void artificially created in you by that first cigarette, not realizing that far from filling the void it temporarily tops it up and then goes on to create a new void.

To take deliberately any drug that interferes with the natural functioning of the most sophisticated object on the planet would be as stupid as altering the calibration of an instrument that was perfectly calibrated. Be absolutely clear: you don't need to smoke, and:

YOU DON'T NEED ANYTHING IN ITS PLACE

This conveniently leads us back to the questionnaire, and Illusion 16: Does it help to use nicotine gum, patches or sprays? Let me now explain exactly why:

ALL SUBSTITUTES MAKE IT HARDER TO STOP

22 *All Substitutes Make It Harder To Stop*

What we are achieving is never to have the need or desire to smoke another cigarette. You might still believe that it is difficult to obtain that state. I promise you that it is simplicity itself, providing you follow all the instructions. It doesn't depend on luck. On the contrary, you will be in complete control.

One of the instructions is not to use any substitutes whatsoever. I have emphasized the importance of removing the belief that you are incomplete or somehow lacking a vital ingredient if you don't smoke. If you search for a substitute, what you are actually saying to yourself is: 'I know smoking is ruining my health and wealth and I'd like to be rid of that side of it; but it was also my pleasure and support and I need something to take its place.' But, by saying this, you are simply confirming that you believe that you are dependent upon the drug. Why else would you need something to take its place?

When you recover from a bout of flu, do you search for another disease to take its place? Of course you don't; you are just happy to know that you are over it. Now re-read the definition of DEVASTATION in Chapter 6; that's the disease you've been suffering from. Now I know you probably still find it difficult to see smoking exactly in those terms, but I aim to convince you. Picture an alcoholic who has descended to the depths of 'skid row'. Everyone can see clearly that, no matter what problems made him turn to alcohol in the first place, by far his worst problem is the alcohol itself, which is providing him with no benefit whatsoever. The one person who cannot see the true situation is, of course, the person who is afflicted. All addictive drugs have this effect on their victims. The more they drag you down (and I'm not talking about the physical effects; those we can see clearly), the more they destroy your courage and confidence, and the greater your need for your illusory friend and support.

It takes imagination to visualize yourself in such a position. It takes courage to use your imagination. So what! Mother Nature has equipped you with imagination and courage, if that's what it takes. We are all a little like the Lion in The Wizard of Oz; we have lost touch with the natural courage and confidence we once had. You are about to find it again.

The quicker you can starve the 'little monster' the better, so the quicker you can remove the 'big monster' the better. Fortunately, the 'big monster' is purely a figment of your imagination, an illusion. Like the world depicted in the film The Matrix, it is a bubble of illusion, and it can be removed before you put out your final cigarette.

All substitutes do is to prolong the life of the bubble. If you don't remove the illusion before you put out the final cigarette, how can you possibly remove it afterwards? All substitutes by design prolong the life of the 'big monster'. Substitutes that contain nicotine have the added disadvantage of prolonging the life of the 'little monster', too. I am, of course, referring to nicotine gum, patches and nasal sprays. Now I know they sound logical. The theory is that when you attempt to 'give up' smoking, you have two powerful adversaries to defeat. The first is the terrible physical pains caused by withdrawal from nicotine; the second is the habit itself. Isn't it just common sense that, if you have two powerful opponents to defeat, only a fool would attempt to take them both on at the same time?

So, the rational theory is that when you put out what you hope will be your final cigarette, while you are breaking the habit and to avoid the terrible physical withdrawal symptoms, you keep your body supplied with nicotine. Having broken the habit, you can now face the second adversary, and ease the problem by gradually cutting down on the intake of nicotine.

It all sounds so plausible, doesn't it? Until you start to scratch the surface. Couldn't exactly the same outcome be achieved simply by gradually cutting down on your smoking? In fact, wouldn't that be even easier? After all, you could further ease the situation by gradually breaking the habit as well as the physical withdrawal pains. Do you remember Mary in Chapter 13? She tried that route and found that, far from removing her illusion of dependence, it simply ingrained into her mind that the most precious thing in life is a cigarette.

Nicotine Replacement Therapy (NRT) sounds logical but it is based on three false assumptions:

1. That smoking is a habit.

2. That habits are difficult to break.

3. That the withdrawal of nicotine creates severe physical withdrawal pains.

We have already exploded all three of these assumptions. You might have noticed that the most common comment of smokers who tried the 'patch' and failed was, 'It definitely helped with the physical withdrawal, but didn't solve the psychological problem.' In other words, it got credit for solving a problem that didn't actually exist, but did nothing to aid the real problem.

I have asked literally dozens of qualified doctors to offer a scientific explanation as to why gradually cutting down cannot provide exactly the same effect as NRT. And why, when it is a proven fact that gradually cutting down makes it ten times harder to stop, they claim that NRT makes it easier. Not one of them has attempted to offer a scientific explanation. I have asked the same doctors, 'How is it possible to help cure a drug addict by prescribing the same drug that the victim is addicted to?' Not only has not one of them attempted to offer an explanation, but it hadn't even occurred to any of them that that was what they were actually doing!

To advise a smoker not to smoke but to chew gum containing nicotine is equivalent to advising a heroin addict not to smoke heroin because smoking is dangerous, but instead to inject it straight into a vein! Even the phrase 'Nicotine Replacement Therapy' is a misnomer. There is no therapy involved and there isn't any replacement. It consists only of prescribing the same drug in a different form. And this is why we have literally thousands of ex-smokers attend our centres in order to be released from addiction to nicotine gum.

So what are we searching for when we seek a substitute? Something that has all the advantages of smoking without the downside? A 'magic' pill that will relieve boredom and improve concentration, that is both a stimulant and a relaxant? Come on! Do you still believe in fairies? Isn't that why you fell into the trap in the first place? As Dorothy discovered: the Wizard of Oz was a fraud. What she was searching for she already had. So do you. Your body combined with your brain doesn't need outside help. They won't eliminate genuine stress, any more than a cigarette will, but they will ensure you get adrenaline on demand to enable you to cope with stress, and they will provide dopamines to relax you and make you feel happy when the danger has passed.

Let's spare a thought for those doctors. A general practitioner not only has to prescribe a cure that will help smokers to stop, but is expected to know the solution to every other disease that might afflict the most sophisticated object on the planet. Let's not be too hard on them. It took me a lifetime to uncover the mysteries of the smoking trap. As with all other diseases, doctors tend to prescribe the solutions that the drug manufacturing conglomerates advocate. The average general practitioner knows no more about nicotine addiction than 'Joe Public'. In fact, we have more medics seek the help of our centres than those of any other profession. I emphasize that they seek it, and it's not to serve their patients better, but to escape from the trap themselves!

So, we are left with just the four final illusions on the questionnaire:

Does it take willpower to stop?

Is it necessary to suffer from physical withdrawal symptoms?

Do ex-smokers have to endure an initial period of craving and irritability?

Is it difficult to stop?

We have already partially addressed all four points. The answer to them all is an emphatic 'No', provided you have followed all the instructions.

You have now reached an exciting stage. Imagine you are Edmund Hillary or Sherpa Tenzing, just a hundred feet from the summit of Everest. All the hard work of your planning and preparation is behind you. The weather is being kind and you know that nothing can prevent you from achieving your goal.

Do you feel a little nervous and anxious? Don't worry about that. Think of Nelson Mandela when they came to open his prison door. Can you imagine the excitement? Do you think he didn't have butterflies in his stomach? You are in a very similar position to Hillary and Tenzing, only better. You don't have to rely on Lady Luck or any other contingencies. You are in exactly the same situation as Mandela. All you need do is to follow:

THE FINAL INSTRUCTIONS

23 *The Final Instructions*

Before we proceed with the final instructions, there is one important subject that we haven't discussed: TIMING. You may be asking yourself, 'Is now really the right time to attempt to stop?'

Please don't fall into that ingenious trap. It will have you thinking there is never a right time. After all, smokers smoke at the most enjoyable times: it would be silly to 'give up' before the wedding, Christmas or the vacation. And then there's the stress: 'I'll wait until I'm feeling more relaxed, and X, Y or Z problem has been resolved.' That kind of thinking sucks us in until it kills us. There is always some celebration or tragedy to persuade us to put off the 'evil' day.

Supposing someone was suffering from a disease that would get progressively worse and there was a simple and inexpensive cure to that disease. When would you advise them to apply the cure? You don't even have to think about it. The answer is, and always has been, NOW! NOW! NOW! What sort of idiot would you have thought Hillary if, having got to within 100 feet of the summit, he had started wondering about his next move, and finally said: 'Perhaps I should wait until next year.'

Nothing bad is happening. On the contrary, something marvellous is happening:

GO FOR IT!

You have had a set of instructions to follow while reading the book. There's no point in repeating them at this stage. However, before you proceed with the ritual of the final cigarette, it is imperative that you fully understand the vital cornerstone on which Easyway is based: that smoking gives you no genuine pleasure or support, in any shape or form. Let me make it absolutely clear: I do not mean that the disadvantages of being a smoker far outweigh any advantages. Every smoker knows this before they become hooked, throughout the time they are hooked and after they have 'given up', even though they continue to crave cigarettes. I mean there are no advantages.

The illusion of pleasure and/or support is created by the fact that when nicotine leaves your body it creates an empty, insecure feeling, an imbalance, and that far from relieving boredom and stress, or aiding relaxation and concentration, smoking does the complete opposite:

NICOTINE CREATED THAT IMBALANCE AND WILL CONTINUE TO RE-CREATE IT ALL THE WHILE YOU FIND AN EXCUSE TO LIGHT JUST ONE MORE CIGARETTE

You need to understand that this scenario applies to every smoker, and not just to you. Unless you are clear about these two points, I would advise you to re-read the book and not to attempt to stop until you are. If you continue to find difficulty, you can obtain further assistance from any Easyway centre (see the listing at the back of the book).

We also need to clear up the final four illusions on the questionnaire:

17. Does it take willpower to stop?

18. Is it necessary to suffer from physical withdrawal symptoms?

19. Do ex-smokers have to endure an initial period of craving and irritability?

20. Is it difficult to stop?

We have already addressed all four points at various stages, and provided you have understood the trap completely, you will know that they are all illusions. Ideally, you should now be like a dog straining at the leash, impatient to smoke that final cigarette and be free. However, if you have tried to stop in the past and found it difficult or impossible, as I did many times, you might not readily accept the idea that any smoker can find it easy and enjoyable. This reservation, however, need not prevent you from making the attempt. As with anything, the proof of the pudding is in the eating – and some people need to eat the pudding first! So, if you feel somewhat nervous and apprehensive, don't worry. Nervous you might be, but you cannot fail to win through, provided you continue to follow all the instructions.

HERE ARE YOUR FINAL INSTRUCTIONS:

1. Check your frame of mind. Remember, the real difference between a smoker and a non-smoker is not that one smokes and the other doesn't. The real difference is that a non-smoker has no need or desire to smoke; not today, not tomorrow, not ever. If you find the thought of never, ever smoking another cigarette difficult to face, try thinking about the alternatives and how they make you feel:

(A) Going through life craving a cigarette but not allowing yourself to have one; or
(B) Never being allowed to stop smoking.

Even if you feel somewhat apprehensive and nervous, this doesn't mean you need to be miserable. It is essential that you start off – and continue – in a happy frame of mind; that you see smoking as it really is (nothing more or less than a drug called DEVASTATION); and that you realize you are about to achieve something marvellous, something that every other smoker on the planet would love to achieve:

RELEASE FROM THE SLAVERY
OF NICOTINE ADDICTION

2. You never decided to become a smoker for life. Like every other smoker, you were lured into the trap. Don't underestimate the ingenuity of that trap. At one time 80 percent of the adult population were imprisoned in it. Unlike someone serving a life sentence in prison, you won't be released after thirty years, and there'll be no remission for good behaviour. This particular prison is designed to keep you enslaved until it kills you. What's worse is that you're being punished for a crime you didn't even commit. You won't escape just by hoping that someday you'll be released by some miracle. The first thing you must do is to make a positive decision to escape.

You are about to do that right now. Some decisions are difficult to make. If you are buying a new car, there are myriad factors to consider. However, the decision you are about to make is probably the most important of your life. You probably think that I am over-dramatising the situation. Like thousands of other smokers who have stopped thanks to Easyway, in hindsight you will realize that the decision you have made today will affect the quality of every other aspect of your life. Bear in mind that the decision you are making is not whether to stop smoking. You have the wonderful choice of deciding whether you spend the rest of your life in the trap or being free of it. Don't kid yourself that if you don't stop today, you'll do it tomorrow. You'll simply be proving my point that the trap has beaten you, and you'll remain imprisoned for life. Fortunately, stopping smoking is not only the most important and beneficial decision you'll ever make, but also the easiest. The beautiful truth is that there are no pros or cons to weigh up. There are no advantages whatsoever to being a smoker. The disadvantages are so hideous that, once hooked, we cannot bear even to think about them. Nevertheless, I want you to make a solemn vow now: that when you have completed the ritual of smoking the final cigarette, no matter what happens in your life, you will never smoke another cigarette.

Having made what you know to be the correct decision, never, ever question or doubt your decision. We've been brainwashed from birth to see smoking as a pleasure and/or support. Be aware that smoking is nothing more or less than addiction to nicotine, and that nicotine is nothing more or less than a drug called DEVASTATION. Your perception of smoking has been distorted. It can become so again. But the facts have never altered. Smoking always was addiction to DEVASTATION, and always will be.

Some smokers find it difficult, if not impossible, to believe that all smokers can find it both easy and enjoyable to stop. Let me emphasize that, although thousands of ex-smokers believe that Easyway works like magic, it isn't magic. It's easy to escape from the most complicated maze, provided you have a map. Many critics believe that Easyway is simply a set of useful tips. It's more than that: it's the map that will enable any smoker to find it easy to stop. The beautiful truth is that it is easy to stop provided you follow the instructions. Smokers only find it difficult to stop because:

(A) They believe they are being deprived of a genuine pleasure and/or support. Because of this:
(B) They put out their final cigarette hoping they will never smoke another and spend the next few days, and the rest of their lives, craving a cigarette and feeling deprived and miserable because they won't allow themselves to have one.

The only difficulty is the doubt, the uncertainty, the waiting for nothing to happen. If you were to follow only one of the instructions, the most important would be to know you had made the right decision and as a consequence never punish yourself by questioning that decision. Then you would find it easy to stop. You would not:

(A) Feel deprived rather than elated at no longer being a smoker.
(B) Envy rather than pity smokers when they light up.

If you don't feel you have made the right decision, you are placing yourself in an impossible position: you'll be moping for and envying a situation that never existed, and cannot exist. You now leave yourself with only two choices. The first is to resist the temptation and feel miserable and deprived. The second is not to resist the temptation and to smoke just one cigarette. You will know for certain that if you can't resist the temptation once, you won't be able to resist it again, and again. You'll still be a slave to nicotine and you'll feel even more miserable.

EITHER WAY YOU'LL BE A LOSER

Fortunately, you do have a third choice. It is to accept that you've been brainwashed. You might find yourself envying other smokers or even fancying a cigarette on occasions, perhaps because you have sat in a smoky atmosphere and have passively taken in nicotine, which may cause a physical reaction. Or you might simply be amazed that those around you seem so content being smokers, and you find yourself thinking they must get something out of it. This is an important warning signal: it means the conditioning and brainwashing are starting to take effect. Remember, the tobacco companies pay with blood money to get into your mind. But you have a defence against their insidious propaganda: you can see that it is all part of the ingenuity of the trap, and one of the many features that keep other nicotine addicts enslaved until they are destroyed. Rejoice in the fact that you now understand just how ingenious the trap is, and that you have already achieved what every smoker on the planet would dearly love to achieve. Instead of allowing such moments to create doubt in your mind, use them to remind yourself of:

HOW MARVELLOUS IT IS TO BE FREE THAT YOU DON'T HAVE TO ENDURE A PERIOD OF TRAUMA THAT YOU DON'T HAVE TO WAIT TO BECOME A NON-SMOKER

If you are waiting, what you are really waiting for is the uncertainty and doubts to disappear. What is there to wait for? Like me, and every other smoker, you know instinctively that smoking is a fool's game. It really is as simple as this: you are about to experience something wonderful:

THE RITUAL OF YOUR FINAL CIGARETTE

If this expression still fills you with apprehension, be aware that it is because you are apprehensive that you will miss smoking and will be unable to enjoy life or cope without it. That is a genuine fear, but one that you didn't have before you fell into the trap.

So let's see the ritual of this final cigarette in its true light. You have been in training for this moment all of your smoking life: to put out a cigarette.

You've set out to achieve something that society in general believes to be very difficult and which many smokers are certain is impossible. Having got this far, you are not even 100 feet from the summit. You have already completed the course. The ritual of the final cigarette is rather like the pomp and circumstance of the Oscar ceremony. Would an Oscar be quite so important without the ceremony? Would a wedding or a funeral be quite the same without the ceremony?

Hillary and Tenzing were alone, but do you think that detracted from the ceremony of planting that flag? The whole world knew of their achievement. Your family, friends, colleagues and acquaintances will shortly know what you have achieved. Don't see it as the ritual of the final cigarette, but as it really is: a ceremony dedicated to you for your personal glorification to celebrate your release and escape from a nightmarish slavery:

NICOTINE ADDICTION

For those of you who have followed my instructions and have continued to smoke until this point, I would like you to smoke your final cigarette now. If you are one of those readers who had already vowed never to smoke another cigarette before you started this book, don't feel that you need to miss out on the ceremony. You have already smoked your final cigarette, but this does not prevent you from celebrating your achievement. In fact it is essential that you do so now, even though you are already ahead of the game. In your case the 'little monster' is either in his final death throes or indeed may already be dead.

It's a pity that we can't hire the Hollywood Bowl and have all the smokers who manage to escape in a given year to attend and celebrate their achievement. I'm convinced that if it were possible to do this with the same publicity that attends the Oscar ceremonies, the inevitable death of nicotine addiction in our society would be hastened.

You can of course complete the ceremony in the company of your close family and friends. You might, however, for whatever reason, prefer to complete it in private.

Whatever your choice, be conscious of smoking that final cigarette. Be aware that there is nothing pleasurable about the taste and that there is something decidedly unpleasureable about breathing bad, cancerous fumes into your lungs. Also be aware that if you choose to go through that ceremony alone, your close family and friends will still be rooting for you.

In fact, although they might not admit it, every smoker on the planet will be rooting for you, because every time someone like you manages to escape from the tyranny, it gives hope to those left in its grips.

I began by stating that no smoker living or dead ever enjoyed smoking a cigarette. I wish to temper that statement. It is possible not only to enjoy smoking one cigarette but to be filled with ecstasy by smoking just one cigarette, provided of course that you understand that it is your last cigarette!

Whether or not you have been straining at the leash, you are now free to release yourself and never to have to suffer the indignity of being restrained or imprisoned again. Please smoke that final cigarette and enjoy turning the key that will release you from:

SLAVERY TO NICOTINE

When you have put out that final cigarette, be aware that you are already a non-smoker. All you need to do from this point on is to accept that smokers, just like non-smokers and ex-smokers, have good days and bad days. In fact, as the addiction drags them further and further down, the good days tend to be fewer and farther between. Expect to feel somewhat disorientated for a few days, but don't worry about it: that's simply a sign that you are recovering. It's really as simple as this: you don't need me to tell you that smokers are fools. All you need to do from this point on, whenever you think about smoking, whether you are having a good day or a bad day, is not to question your decision, but to get into the habit of thinking:

YIPPEE, I'M A NON-SMOKER!

This isn't just a mantra: by repeating something you hope it becomes the truth. It is the truth. The ingenuity of the trap has conditioned you to believe that any empty, insecure feeling can be partly relieved by smoking a cigarette. The whole purpose of Easyway is to help you understand that the complete opposite is the truth. It takes time to adjust to this truth. In the meantime, just follow all the instructions and, if you haven't already experienced it, in a few days you will soon enjoy a wonderful experience. I call it the 'Moment of Revelation'. This is similar to the feeling you get when you swim for the first time without water wings or other aids, or when you pass your driving test. When you become a fully qualified driver, the world is your oyster. You can go anywhere you want to without having to beg some unfortunate to risk their life accompanying you. You are self-reliant, as when you finally learnt to ride that two-wheeler bike without stabilizers or a parental hand to hold you steady. This has been beautifully epitomized in a TV ad: a young boy keeps repeating, 'Don't let go, Dad'; he looks round and realizes that Dad has already let go and that he has ridden 50 yards unaided and in control.

The real joy of these moments comes out of the achiever's sense of a new-found freedom, and that they are no longer dependent on someone else.

The 'Moment of Revelation' far exceeds any of the examples I have given. It's nice not to be dependent on people who love you and are only too happy to help you. To realize that you are no longer dependent on a filthy poison that you know is killing you, to be free of the self-despising that comes with knowing you are paying a fortune to be a slave to a poison, that is something else. It is a special moment.

This special moment usually occurs a few days after you have stopped, after one of those situations that you thought you couldn't enjoy or handle without a cigarette. It could be a party you attended or a stressful situation you coped with. Afterwards it dawns on you: not only didn't you smoke to get you through, but you never even thought about smoking. Then you realize that everything I've been saying is true: social occasions can be more pleasant, you are better equipped to handle stress, you don't have to spend the rest of your life feeling that you are missing out, and the expression 'once a smoker always a smoker' is bunkum.

Just as trying not to think about smoking will create a phobia and guarantee that you'll never stop thinking about it, so trying to create the 'Moment of Revelation' will guarantee that you never achieve it. Smokers using a 'willpower' method rarely have that Moment of Revelation, because they are never sure they have succeeded. If your objective is to stop smoking for a week or a year, you cannot possibly know that you have succeeded in your goal until the week or year has passed. On the same basis, if your objective is never to smoke again, you won't know whether or not you have succeeded until your life is over. In effect, you will never know.

So how will you know with Easyway? Because you understand the nature of the trap. Fish in a shoal might compete to be the first to swallow a piece of bait, but the fish that knows that the bait conceals a hook won't be tempted even to nibble at it; that fish will just pity the others, and particularly the winner of the competition.

You are already a non-smoker. The nightmare is over. The main objective of this book wasn't to help you to stop smoking. It was to enable you to enjoy life more. Get on and do just that.

A small minority of ex-smokers find it relatively easy to stop with Easyway and are quite happy to remain non-smokers, but do not experience the 'Moment of Revelation'. This is because they have failed to follow all of the instructions. You might remember Fiona's case in Chapter 14:

'I understand and agree with everything you say in Easyway. Let me make it clear that I'm deliriously happy to be a non-smoker and know that I will never smoke again. I know you say that whenever I think about smoking it must be: "Isn't it great! I'm free!" and that's how I genuinely feel all the time, except when I open the front door to that empty house. I can't help thinking: "if only I could have just one cigarette." I know it won't only be one cigarette so I don't have it. But I've been free for six months now. Can you please help me?'

When I met Fiona, I pointed out that she must have missed or misunderstood something I 'd said. We discovered that she hadn't broken the association between that sad moment of entering her empty house and the illusory comfort of lighting a cigarette. What she was doing was making that sad moment even sadder by moping for something that she wouldn't allow herself to have, particularly as it wouldn't solve the real problem, which was the empty house and her sense of solitude. We discussed her situation in more depth and she readily accepted that entering the empty house was for her a genuinely sad moment, there being no one inside to share the trials and tribulations of the day. As a naturally gregarious person, she felt saddened by her situation. How many cigarettes would it take to alter the true position? She re-read her personal statement.

This confirmed that she was sick to death of the house being empty and of sitting there alone, smoking away, poisoning herself and not living her life to the full. We humans seldom praise ourselves for our achievements, and are constantly seeking to do better next time. Fiona's case underlines how essential it is to re-write your thoughts and patterns of behaviour so that when the bell tolls it won't be for you! The moment Fiona decided that opening that door each evening could be used as a reminder of just how nice it was to have gained control of something she despised, and that she could cope, the result was a revelation, to both of us. She wrote:

'I did what you suggested from Monday to Thursday and I was fine. I was dreading Friday because that was usually the worst night – a whole weekend in an empty house! The amazing thing was, when I entered the house I didn't even think about how nice it was not to have to smoke. But even more amazing, I was actually looking forward to being home! And it wasn't just because I now felt completely free of the smoking. It dawned on me that I'd been treating my divorce in exactly the same way as my smoking. Excuse my language, but he was a selfish, inconsiderate bastard! Before I fell in love with him and married him, I was happy and confident. I don't wish to brag, but I was never short of boyfriends. He sapped all my confidence, made my life a misery and left me a nervous wreck. Like the smoking, I'd been moping for a situation that never existed.'

The letter went on rather like Debbie's. I don't wish to take credit for situations for which I am not responsible, but quitting smoking is regarded as an incredibly difficult goal to achieve. Once you achieve it, the confidence and belief in yourself that it inspires enables you to confront and control aspects of your life that previously caused you concern. I believe this to be the greatest of the many advantages that being free of nicotine confers.

I experienced the 'Moment of Revelation' before I put out my final cigarette. At our centres, some smokers experience it long before the therapy is complete. They'll say something like: 'You needn't say another word. I can see it all so clearly. Smoking is

just a giant confidence trick and I know I'll never smoke again.'
Possibly you too have already experienced it. Don't worry if you
haven't. Many different factors can affect the situation: the degree
of despondency the drug has reduced you to; whether you have a
good imagination or have to wait for the 'proof of the pudding';
and, most important of all, whether you are just a sheep to be
led along any path, no matter how nonsensical, or are capable of
opening your mind to accept the truth. It doesn't matter if you
score poorly on all counts. If you have followed all the instructions,
you will already be a happy non-smoker. You might once have
thought it was impossible to be a happy ex-smoker. When you
experience the 'Moment of Revelation', you'll find it difficult to
believe that you could ever fall into the trap again. Please read the
final chapter to discover:

HOW TO REMAIN A HAPPY NON-SMOKER FOR THE REST OF YOUR LIFE

24 *How To Remain A Happy Non-smoker For The Rest Of Your Life*

When I reached the 'Moment of Revelation' I knew I could never again fall into the nicotine trap. Several decades later nothing has happened to change this belief, except to reinforce it. I also believed that every other smoker who found it easy to escape with the help of Easyway would be just as invulnerable. A few months later I discovered this was not necessarily so and suffered my biggest setback. Imagine my embarassment when Emma Freud asked for her Introduction to my Easyway video to be removed.

I was pleased to comply with the request. No matter how proud I was of that Introduction, or how many smokers it had helped to escape, the last thing I wanted was a recommendation by someone who had started smoking again. I'd already learned that when my method is recommended by someone who has started smoking again, the smoker receiving the recommendation says one thing and thinks another. The words coming out might be: 'Oh, really? You left that centre after just four hours and were already a happy non-smoker, and it cost less than £150/$198? That must be the best deal of your life! I'll definitely give it a try!' However, what they will be thinking is: 'What sort of fool do you think I am? If it was so easy and enjoyable, why did you start again?'

Why indeed? Since I first discovered Easyway I've spent more time puzzling over this particular aspect of smoking than all the other aspects combined. Of course a cynic would take the attitude: 'Lots of people have managed to abstain for varying periods and were quite happy to be non-smokers. But they weren't really free and eventually they started smoking again. They'd just been kidding themselves!' I'm not ashamed to admit that, were it not I who had discovered Easyway, my attitude would have been exactly the same. No way would I have squandered that sum of money, no matter how vehemently the ex-smoker had praised the method.

My pondering hasn't been completely unproductive. I know and have to accept that a small percentage of smokers will fail to stop for three months. I take considerable pride in having reduced that percentage from 24 percent in my initial year, to less than 5 percent in my latest year. I know also that by far the biggest tragedy with Easyway is not failure to succeed initially, but succeeding and then getting hooked again. I have every reason to believe that I have substantially reduced this percentage too, but unfortunately it has not been possible for me to acquire accurate statistics. This final chapter is an attempt to ensure that you don't become one of those statistics.

I claim that Easyway can not only enable any smoker to find it easy to stop, but to do so permanently. How can I make such a claim and at the same time admit that there will always be a percentage of smokers who will succeed initially but get hooked again? Many will declare that you can't claim to have stopped permanently if you get hooked again. True, but you can claim that you were released from a bear trap and are now completely free. It is also possible to step into another bear trap at a later date. Does that mean you weren't released from the first trap?

I've already expounded on the fact that with a 'willpower' method ex-smokers aren't completely free and remain vulnerable for the rest of their lives. With Easyway you are free the moment the brainwashing has been reversed. Consider the case of Doris, one of the first visitors to our Birmingham centre. She arrived in tears, and about as depressed as it is possible for a smoker to get. She also left in tears; tears of joy, I hasten to add, which spread to the remainder of the centre, including me. She gave me a big kiss as she departed in a state of euphoria, already a happy non-smoker. She visited her daughter and son-in-law the same evening to inform them of the good news. He had promised to 'give up' at the same time, not because he wanted to, but just to support his mother-in-law. But, of course, he was using the 'willpower' method and his mother-in-law's obvious delight only served to increase his feeling of deprivation. He said, 'Why are you getting so excited? You haven't even stopped for a day!' The effect was catastrophic. The four hours I had spent helping that lady out of the pit were destroyed in a couple of seconds. So much for his support. She didn't smoke in their presence, but the seed of doubt had been planted. It germinated, festered and grew.

When Doris left the centre, she was already a happy non-smoker and set to remain one for the rest of her life. You might argue that she had little hope of remaining free if just a few words were all it took to get her hooked again. But she did remain free. Fortunately, she came back to see me. I reminded her of the battle that rages between smokers and ex-smokers, that she should put herself in her son-in-law's position. He was not deliberately trying to undermine her. He was simply defending himself. There she was ecstatic that she no longer had to smoke. But there he was depressed and miserable because he had to 'give up'. She couldn't wait to get back and hit him with her Royal Straight Flush, and that's exactly what she did.

You are free from the moment the brainwashing is removed and you adopt the right frame of mind. But never become blasé. If Easyway has a weakness it is this: because it makes stopping so easy, clients can become over-confident. One of the kindnesses of Mother Nature is that generally she allows us to remember the good times and forget the tragedies. Unfortunately, this can backfire on us. By the end of the course the smoker knows there are many powerful and valid reasons never to smoke again, and not a single valid reason to continue. But over time the bad side of smoking is forgotten. The danger isn't so much in the early days when you are apprehensive and can remember how much you hated being a smoker. The reason I wanted you to record your 'Personal Record' was so that you could refer to it occasionally and remind yourself of exactly why it is great to be free. Make sure you record your feelings when you receive the 'Moment of Revelation'.

Whenever I'm in contact with a smoker who stopped for an extended period but started smoking again, I always ask them: 'Did you enjoy being a non-smoker while you were free?' Without a single exception, the reply is along the lines of: 'It was wonderful!' This is followed by a description of how wonderful it was. I then ask them if they enjoy being a smoker again. Without a single exception, the reply is something like: 'I hate it! Why was I so stupid?' I get exactly the same response from smokers who succeeded for a time using a 'willpower' method. Please learn from their mistakes. If it happens to a client who has already sent me a letter similar to Debbie's, the problem is usually solved simply by returning their letter to them, to remind them of how they felt when they stopped.

Why was the knowledge that Emma had started smoking again such a blow? After all, she was young, healthy and wealthy and had less reason to stop. She was also engaged in a highly stressful and competitive profession in which temptation is rife. It was because she was so obviously highly intelligent, but also probably the nicest person I've had the privilege to meet. As well as being a successful role model to young girls, being a descendant of the great Sigmund added considerable power to her elbow. She was not wrong to ask for her Introduction to be removed. She must have felt a hypocrite and probably suffered great embarrassment from the remarks of her friends who knew that she had started smoking again.

I have nothing but respect for Emma and bear her no ill-will. However, I do despise myself for agreeing to remove her Introduction. If I've learned one lesson in this life, it is that honesty is the best policy; not for moral or idealistic reasons, but for the purely selfish reason that it pays. I should have insisted that the Introduction remained. It was quite obvious that Emma was being honest and sincere and at that time genuinely enjoyed being a happy non-smoker. I should have used that Introduction as a warning, as I'm doing now.

It is easy to stop immediately and permanently, but never underestimate the ingenuity of the trap. You have made a solemn vow never, ever to smoke another cigarette.

The most important instruction of Easyway is: having made what you know to be the correct decision, never, ever doubt or question that decision.

Whenever you think about smoking from now on and for the rest of your life, just remind yourself:

YIPPEE, I'M A NON-SMOKER!

That way you won't even have to use willpower to resist breaking your vow. The important point I'm making is that just as initial success is guaranteed, provided you follow all the instructions, so permanent success is guaranteed. Any smoker who fails to stop initially or permanently with Easyway does so not because Easyway didn't work for them, but because they failed to follow all the instructions.

Let's use Fiona as a final example. She failed to follow just one instruction: to remove all the associations. However, she was still deliriously happy to be a non-smoker and knew that she would never smoke again. But how could she or I know that for certain without removing the remaining piece of brainwashing? The answer is that we can't. All we know is that once that piece of brainwashing was removed, she felt completely free in every aspect of her life. How do we know that there is not some other aspect of Easyway that Fiona, or you for that matter, has missed. We don't, but as they say: 'If it ain't broke, don't waste your time and money trying to fix it.' However, if you do have a problem, either now or in the future, just refer to The Principal Instructions to Follow While Reading This Book.

Read through them now. Don't just skip over each item, thinking: 'Yes, that's obvious.' You have worked so hard getting this far. For the sake of a few extra minutes, it would be a shame to ruin it all by being blasé. Treat each item seriously. Ask yourself: do I really believe this point? Do I really understand it? If you do that for me, I can do no more than repeat Emma's words:

HAVE FUN!

The Principal Instructions To Follow While Reading This Book

The Instructions To Follow That Make It Easy To Stop Permanently

1. Keep this book safely in a place where you can easily refer to it. Do not lose it, lend it out or give it away.

2. Never forget that smoking confers no advantages whatsoever on you or any other smoker.

3. Never envy other smokers. They'll be envying you. You are not being deprived. They are.

4. Having made what you know to be the correct decision, never question or doubt it.

5. Be aware that the 'little monster' will survive for a few days and that you might find yourself reaching for a cigarette. If this happens, don't worry about it. Use the moment to remind yourself just how nice it is to be free.

6. Enjoy breaking the associations. Make a point of finding them to destroy them.

7. Don't use substitutes – you don't need them.

8. Accept that you'll have good days and bad, but never forget that the good days will be better and the bad days less so and fewer.

9. Don't avoid smoking situations or change your lifestyle just because you've stopped smoking, unless you wish to change it for purely selfish reasons. Remember: you've only stopped smoking, not living!

10. Do not attempt to cut down or to control your intake.

11. Re-read your 'personal statement'. Put it on your computer as a screensaver.

12. Ignore the advice of 'experts' and friends if it contradicts these instructions, no matter how eminent these people are or how impressive they sound.

13. Don't wait for the 'Moment of Revelation' or to become a non-smoker – you are already one. Just get on with your life.

14. If you have any difficulties contact your nearest Allen Carr centre. You will find a list of these on the following pages.

15. Above all, don't try not to think about smoking. Whenever you do, tell yourself:

YIPPEE, I'M A NON-SMOKER!

Final Warning

You can now enjoy the rest of your life as a happy non-smoker. In order to make sure that you do, you need to follow these simple instructions.

1. Keep this book safely in a place where you can easily refer to it. Do not lose it, lend it out or give it away.

2. If you ever start to envy another smoker, realize that they will be envious of you. You are not being deprived. They are.

3. Remember you did not enjoy being a smoker. That's why you stopped. You do enjoy being a non-smoker.

4. Remember, there is no such thing as just one cigarette.

5. Never doubt your decision never to smoke again. You know it's the correct decision.

6. If you have any difficulties, contact your nearest Allen Carr centre. You will find a list of these on the following pages.

ALLEN CARR'S EASYWAY CENTRES

The following list indicates the countries where Allen Carr's Easyway To Stop Smoking Centres are currently operational.

Check www.allencarr.com for latest additions to this list.

The success rate at the centres, based on the three-month, money-back guarantee, is over 90 percent.

Selected centres also offer sessions that deal with alcohol, other drugs and weight issues. Please check with your nearest centre, listed below, for details.

Allen Carr's Easyway guarantee that you will find it easy to stop at the centres or your money back.

JOIN US!

Allen Carr's Easyway Centres have spread throughout the world with incredible speed and success. Our global franchise network now covers more than 150 cities in over 45 countries. This amazing growth has been achieved entirely organically. Former addicts, just like you, were so impressed by the ease with which they stopped that they felt inspired to contact us to see how they could bring the method to their region.

If you feel the same, contact us for details on how to become an Allen Carr's Easyway To Stop Smoking or an Allen Carr's Easyway To Stop Drinking franchisee.

Email us at: **join-us@allencarr.com** including your full name, postal address and region of interest.

SUPPORT US!

No, don't send us money!

You have achieved something really marvellous. Every time we hear of someone escaping from the sinking ship, we get a feeling of enormous satisfaction.

It would give us great pleasure to hear that you have freed yourself from the slavery of addiction so please visit the following web page where you can tell us of your success, inspire others to follow in your footsteps and hear about ways you can help to spread the word.

www.allencarr.com/fanzone

You can "like" our facebook page here
www.facebook.com/AllenCarr

Together, we can help further Allen Carr's mission: to cure the world of addiction.

LONDON CENTRE AND WORLDWIDE HEAD OFFICE

Park House, 14 Pepys Road, Raynes Park, London SW20 8NH
Tel: +44 (0)20 8944 7761
Fax: +44 (0)20 8944 8619
Email: mail@allencarr.com
Website: www.allencarr.com
Therapists: John Dicey, Colleen Dwyer, Crispin Hay, Emma Hudson, Rob Fielding, Sam Kelser, Sam Cleary, Rob Groves

Worldwide Press Office

Contact: John Dicey
Tel: +44 (0)7970 88 44 52
Email: media@allencarr.com

UK Centre Information and Central Booking Line

Tel: 0800 389 2115 (UK only)

USA

Denver

Toll free: 1 866 666 4299 /
New York: 212-330 9194
Therapists: Damian O'Hara, Collene Curran, David Skeist
Email: info@theeasywaytostopsmoking.com
Website: www.allencarr.com

Houston

Toll free: 1 866 666 4299 /
New York: 212-330 9194
Therapists: Damian O'Hara, Collene Curran, David Skeist
Email: info@theeasywaytostopsmoking.com
Website: www.allencarr.com

Los Angeles

Toll free: 1 866 666 4299 /
New York: 212-330 9194
Therapists: Damian O'Hara, Collene Curran, David Skeist
Email: info@theeasywaytostopsmoking.com
Website: www.allencarr.com

Milwaukee (and South Wisconsin)

Tel: +1 262 770 1260
Therapist: Wayne Spaulding
Email: wayne@
easywaywisconsin.com
Website: www.allencarr.com

New York

Toll free: 1 866 666 4299 /
New York: 212- 330 9194
Therapists: Damian O'Hara,
Collene Curran, David Skeist
Email: info@
theeasywaytostopsmoking.com
Website: www.allencarr.com

CANADA

Sessions held throughout
Canada
Toll free: +1-866 666 4299 /
+1 905 849 7736
English Therapist:
Damian O'Hara
French Therapist:
Rejean Belanger
Email: info@
theeasywaytostopsmoking.com

Website: www.allencarr.com

UK CENTRES

Birmingham

Tel & Fax: +44 (0)121 423 1227
Therapists: John Dicey,
Colleen Dwyer, Crispin
Hay, Emma Hudson, Rob
Fielding, Sam Kelser, Ania
Martin, Rob Groves
Email: mail@allencarr.com
Website: www.allencarr.com

Brentwood

Tel: 0800 389 2115
Therapists: John Dicey,
Colleen Dwyer, Crispin
Hay, Emma Hudson, Rob
Fielding, Sam Kelser, Rob
Groves
Email: mail@allencarr.com
Website: www.allencarr.com

Brighton

Tel: 0800 389 2115
Therapists: John Dicey,
Colleen Dwyer, Crispin
Hay, Emma Hudson, Rob
Fielding, Sam Kelser, Rob
Groves
Email: mail@allencarr.com
Website: www.allencarr.com

Bristol

Tel: 0800 389 2115
Therapists: John Dicey,
Colleen Dwyer, Crispin Hay,
Emma Hudson, Rob Fielding,
Sam Kelser, Rob Groves
Email: mail@allencarr.com
Website: www.allencarr.com

Cambridge

Tel: 0800 389 2115
Therapists: John Dicey,
Colleen Dwyer, Crispin
Hay, Emma Hudson, Rob
Fielding, Sam Kelser, Rob
Groves
Email: mail@allencarr.com
Website: www.allencarr.com

Coventry

Tel: 0800 321 3007
Therapist: Rob Fielding
Email: info@
easywaymidlands.co.uk
Website: www.allencarr.com

Cumbria

Tel: 0800 077 6187
Therapist: Mark Keen
Email: mark@
easywaymanchester.co.uk
Website: www.allencarr.com

Derby

Tel: 0800 389 2115
Therapist: John Dicey,
Colleen Dwyer, Crispin
Hay, Emma Hudson, Rob
Fielding, Sam Kelser, Rob
Groves
Email: mail@allencarr.com
Website: www.allencarr.com

Guernsey
Tel: 0800 077 6187
Therapist: Mark Keen
Email: mark@
easywaymanchester.co.uk
Website: www.allencarr.com

Isle of Man
Tel: 0800 077 6187
Therapist: Mark Keen
Email: mark@
easywaymanchester.co.uk
Website: www.allencarr.com

Jersey
Tel: 0800 077 6187
Therapist: Mark Keen
Email: mark@
easywaymanchester.co.uk
Website: www.allencarr.com

Kent
Tel: 0800 389 2115
Therapists: John Dicey,
Colleen Dwyer, Crispin
Hay, Emma Hudson, Rob
Fielding, Sam Kelser,
Rob Groves

Email: mail@allencarr.com
Website: www.allencarr.com

Lancashire
Tel: 0800 077 6187
Therapist: Mark Keen
Email: mark@
easywaymanchester.co.uk
Website: www.allencarr.com

Leeds
Tel: 0800 077 6187
Therapist: Mark Keen
Email: mark@
easywaymanchester.co.uk
Website: www.allencarr.com

Leicester
Tel: 0800 321 3007
Therapist: Rob Fielding
Email: info@
easywaymidlands.co.uk
Website: www.allencarr.com

Lincoln

Tel: 0800 321 3007
Therapist: Rob Fielding
Email: info@
easywaymidlands.co.uk
Website: www.allencarr.com

Liverpool

Tel: 0800 077 6187
Therapist: Mark Keen
Email: mark@
easywaymanchester.co.uk
Website: www.allencarr.com

Manchester

Tel: 0800 077 6187
Therapist: Mark Keen
Email: mark@
easywaymanchester.co.uk
Website: www.allencarr.com

Manchester—alcohol sessions

Tel: +44 (0)7936 712942
Therapist: Mike Connolly
Email: info@
stopdrinkingnorth.co.uk
Website: www.allencarr.com

Milton Keynes

Tel: 0800 389 2115
Therapists: John Dicey,
Colleen Dwyer, Crispin
Hay, Emma Hudson, Rob
Fielding, Sam Kelser, Rob
Groves
Email: mail@allencarr.com
Website: www.allencarr.com

Newcastle/North East

Tel: 0800 077 6187
Therapist: Mark Keen
Email: mark@
easywaymanchester.co.uk
Website: www.allencarr.com

Northern Ireland/Belfast

Tel: 0800 077 6187
Therapist: Mark Keen
Email: mark@
easywaymanchester.co.uk
Website: www.allencarr.com

Nottingham

Tel: 0800 389 2115
Therapist: John Dicey,
Colleen Dwyer, Crispin

Hay, Emma Hudson, Rob Fielding, Sam Kelser, Rob Groves
Email: mail@allencarr.com
Website: www.allencarr.com

Reading
Tel: 0800 389 2115
Therapists: John Dicey, Colleen Dwyer, Crispin Hay, Emma Hudson, Rob Fielding, Sam Kelser, Rob Groves
Email: mail@allencarr.com
Website: www.allencarr.com

SCOTLAND
Glasgow and Edinburgh
Tel: +44 (0)131 449 7858
Therapists: Paul Melvin and Jim McCreadie
Email: info@ easywayscotland.co.uk
Website: www.allencarr.com

Southampton
Tel: 0800 389 2115
Therapists: John Dicey, Colleen Dwyer, Crispin Hay, Emma Hudson, Rob Fielding, Sam Kelser, Rob Groves
Email: mail@allencarr.com
Website: www.allencarr.com

Southport
Tel: 0800 077 6187
Therapist: Mark Keen
Email: mark@ easywaymanchester.co.uk
Website: www.allencarr.com

Staines/Heathrow
Tel: 0800 389 2115
Therapists: John Dicey, Colleen Dwyer, Crispin Hay, Emma Hudson, Rob Fielding, Sam Kelser, Rob Groves
Email: mail@allencarr.com
Website: www.allencarr.com

Stevenage

Tel: 0800 389 2115
Therapists: John Dicey,
Colleen Dwyer, Crispin
Hay, Emma Hudson, Rob
Fielding, Sam Kelser, Rob
Groves
Email: mail@allencarr.com
Website: www.allencarr.com

Stoke

Tel: 0800 389 2115
Therapist: John Dicey, Colleen
Dwyer, Crispin Hay, Emma
Hudson, Rob Fielding, Sam
Kelser, Rob Groves
Email: mail@allencarr.com
Website: www.allencarr.com

Surrey

Park House, 14 Pepys Road,
Raynes Park, London
SW20 8NH
Tel: +44 (0)20 8944 7761
Fax: +44 (0)20 8944 8619
Therapists: John Dicey,
Colleen Dwyer, Crispin
Hay, Emma Hudson, Rob

Fielding, Sam Kelser, Rob
Groves, Sam Cleary
Email: mail@allencarr.com
Website: www.allencarr.com

Watford

Tel: 0800 389 2115
Therapists: John Dicey,
Colleen Dwyer, Crispin
Hay, Emma Hudson, Rob
Fielding, Sam Kelser, Rob
Groves
Email: mail@allencarr.com
Website: www.allencarr.com

Worcester

Tel: 0800 321 3007
Therapist: Rob Fielding
Email: info@
easywaymidlands.co.uk
Website: www.allencarr.com

WORLDWIDE CENTRES

REPUBLIC OF IRELAND
Dublin and Cork

Lo-Call (From ROI)
1 890 ESYWAY (37 99 29)

Tel: +353 (0)1 499 9010
(4 lines)
Therapists: Brenda Sweeney
and Team
Email: info@allencarr.ie
Website: www.allencarr.com

AUSTRALIA
ACT, NSW, NT, QSL, VIC
Tel: 1300 848 028
Therapist: Natalie Clays
Email: natalie@
allencarr.com.au
Website: www.allencarr.com

South Australia
Tel: 1300 848 028
Therapist: Jaime Reed
Email: sa@allencarr.com.au
Website: www.allencarr.com

Western Australia
Tel: 1300 848 0281
Therapist: Dianne Fisher
Email: wa@allencarr.com.au
Website: www.allencarr.com

AUSTRIA
Sessions held throughout
Austria
Freephone: 0800RAUCHEN
(0800 7282436)
Tel: +43 (0)3512 44755
Therapists: Erich Kellermann
and Team
Email: info@allen-carr.at
Website: www.allencarr.com

BAHRAIN—opening 2018
Website: www.allencarr.com

BELGIUM
Antwerp
Tel: +32 (0)3 281 6255
Fax: +32 (0)3 744 0608
Therapist: Dirk Nielandt
Email: info@allencarr.be
Website: www.allencarr.com

BRAZIL
São Paulo
Therapists: Alberto Steinberg
& Lilian Brunstein
Email:
contato@easywaysp.com.br

Tel Lilian -
(55) (11)99456-0153
Tel Alberto -
(55) (11)99325-6514
Website: www.allencarr.com

BULGARIA
Tel: 0800 14104 /
+359 899 88 99 07
Therapist: Rumyana
Kostadinova
Email: rk@nepushaveche.com
Website: www.allencarr.com

CHILE
Tel: +56 2 4744587
Therapist: Claudia Sarmiento
Email: contacto@allencarr.cl
Website: www.allencarr.com

CZECH REPUBLIC
Tel: +420 234 261 787
Therapist: Dagmar Janecková
Email: dagmar.janeckova@
allencarr.cz
Website: www.allencarr.com

DENMARK
Sessions held throughout
Denmark
Tel: +45 70267711
Therapist: Mette Fonss
Email: mette@easyway.dk
Website: www.allencarr.com

ESTONIA
Tel: +372 733 0044
Therapist: Henry Jakobson
Email: info@allencarr.ee
Website: www.allencarr.com

FINLAND
Tel: +358-(0)45 3544099
Therapist: Janne Ström
Email: info@allencarr.fi
Website: www.allencarr.com

FRANCE
Sessions held throughout France
Freephone: 0800 386387
Tel: +33 (4)91 33 54 55
Therapists: Erick Serre
and Team
Email: info@allencarr.fr
Website: www.allencarr.com

GERMANY

Sessions held throughout
Germany
Freephone: 08000RAUCHEN
(0800 07282436)
Tel: +49 (0) 8031 90190-0
Therapists: Erich Kellermann
and Team
Email: info@allen-carr.de
Website: www.allencarr.com

GREECE

Sessions held throughout
Greece
Tel: +30 210 5224087
Therapist: Panos Tzouras
Email: panos@allencarr.gr
Website: www.allencarr.com

GUATEMALA

Tel: +502 2362 0000
Therapist: Michelle Binford
Email: bienvenid@
dejedefumarfacil.com
Website: www.allencarr.com

HONG KONG

Email: info@
easywayhongkong.com
Website: www.allencarr.com

HUNGARY

Seminars in Budapest and 12
other cities across Hungary
Tel: 06 80 624 426 (freephone)
or +36 20 580 9244
Therapist: Gabor Szasz
Email: szasz.gabor@
allencarr.hu
Website: www.allencarr.com

ICELAND
Reykjavik

Tel: +354 588 7060
Therapist: Petur Einarsson
Email: easyway@easyway.is
Website: www.allencarr.com

INDIA
Bangalore and Chennai
Tel: +91 (0)80 4154 0624
Therapist: Suresh Shottam
Email: info@
easywaytostopsmoking.co.in
Website: www.allencarr.com

IRAN—opening 2018
Tehran and Mashhad
Website: www.allencarr.com

ISRAEL
Sessions held throughout
Israel
Tel: +972 (0)3 6212525
Therapists:
Ramy Romanovsky,
Orit Rozen
Email: info@allencarr.co.il
Website: www.allencarr.com

ITALY
Sessions held throughout
Italy
Tel/Fax: +39 (0)2 7060 2438
Therapists: Francesca Cesati
and Team

Email: info@
easywayitalia.com
Website: www.allencarr.com

JAPAN
Sessions held throughout
Japan
www.allencarr.com

LEBANON
Tel: +961 1 791 5565
Therapist: Sadek El-Assaad
Email: stopsmoking@
allencarreasyway.me
Website: www.allencarr.com

MAURITIUS
Tel: +230 5727 5103
Therapist: Heidi Hoareau
Email: info@allencarr.mu
Website: www.allencarr.com

MEXICO
Sessions held throughout
Mexico
Tel: +52 55 2623 0631
Therapists: Jorge Davo
Email: info@allencarr-
mexico.com
Website: www.allencarr.com

NETHERLANDS
Sessions held throughout the
Netherlands
Allen Carr's Easyway
'stoppen met roken'
Tel: (+31)53 478 43 62 /
(+31)900 786 77 37
Email: info@allencarr.nl
Website: www.allencarr.com

NEW ZEALAND
North Island – Auckland
Tel: +64 (0)27 4139 381
Therapist: Vickie Macrae
Email: vickie@easywaynz.co.nz
Website: www.allencarr.com

South Island – Dunedin and Invercargill
Tel: +64 (0)27 4139 381
Therapist: Debbie Kinder
Email: easywaysouth@
icloud.com
Website: www.allencarr.com

NORWAY
Oslo
Tel: +47 93 20 09 11
Therapist: René Adde
Email: post@easyway-norge.no
Website: www.allencarr.com

PERU
Lima
Tel: +511 637 7310
Therapist: Luis Loranca
Email: lloranca@
dejardefumaraltoque.com
Website: www.allencarr.com

POLAND

Sessions held throughout
Poland
Tel: +48 (0)22 621 36 11
Therapist: Anna Kabat
Email: info@allen-carr.pl
Website: www.allencarr.com

PORTUGAL
Oporto

Tel: +351 22 9958698
Therapist: Ria Slof
Email: info@
comodeixardefumar.com
Website: www.allencarr.com

ROMANIA

Tel: +40 (0)7321 3 8383
Therapist: Diana Vasiliu
Email: raspunsuri@allencarr.ro
Website: www.allencarr.com

RUSSIA
Moscow

Tel: +7 495 644 64 26
Therapist: Alexander Fomin
Email: info@allencarr.ru
Website: www.allencarr.com

St Petersburg

Website: www.allencarr.com

SAUDI ARABIA—opening 2018

Website: www.allencarr.com

SERBIA
Belgrade

Tel: +381 (0)11 308 8686
Email: office@allencarr.co.rs
Website: www.allencarr.com

SINGAPORE

Tel: +65 62241450
Therapist: Pam Oei
Email: pam@allencarr.com.sg
Website: www.allencarr.com

SLOVAKIA
Tel: +421 233 04 69 92
Therapist: Peter Sánta
Email: peter.santa@allencarr.sk
Website: www.allencarr.com

SLOVENIA
Tel: 00386 (0)40 77 61 77
Therapist: Gregor Server
Email: easyway@easyway.si
Website: www.allencarr.com

SOUTH AFRICA
Sessions held throughout
South Africa
National Booking Line: 0861
100 200
Head Office: 15 Draper
Square, Draper St, Claremont
7708, Cape Town
Cape Town: Dr Charles Nel
Tel: +27 (0)21 851 5883
Mobile: 083 600 5555
Therapists: Dr Charles Nel,
Malcolm Robinson and Team
Email: easyway@allencarr.co.za
Website: www.allencarr.com

SOUTH KOREA
Seoul
Tel: +82 (0)70 4227 1862
Therapist: Yousung Cha
Email: master@allencarr.co.kr
Website: www.allencarr.com

SWEDEN
Tel: +46 70 695 6850
Therapists: Nina Ljungqvist,
Renée Johansson
Email: info@easyway.se
Website: www.allencarr.com

SWITZERLAND
Sessions held throughout
Switzerland
Freephone: 0800RAUCHEN
(0800/728 2436)
Tel: +41 (0)52 383 3773
Fax: +41 (0)52 3833774
Therapists: Cyrill Argast
and Team
For sessions in Suisse
Romand and Svizzera
Italiana: Tel: 0800 386 387
Email: info@allen-carr.ch
Website: www.allencarr.com

TURKEY
Sessions held throughout
Turkey
Tel: +90 212 358 5307
Therapist: Emre Ustunucar
Email: info@
allencarrturkiye.com
Website: www.allencarr.com

UNITED ARAB EMIRATES
Dubai and Abu Dhabi
Tel: +971 56 693 4000
Therapist: Sadek El-Assaad
Email: iwanttoquit@
allencarreasyway.me
Website: www.allencarr.com

OTHER ALLEN CARR PUBLICATIONS

Allen Carr's revolutionary Easyway method is available in a wide variety of formats, including digitally as audiobooks and ebooks, and has been successfully applied to a broad range of subjects.

For more information about Easyway publications, please visit **shop.allencarr.com**

Allen Carr's Quit Smoking Without Willpower

The Only Way to Stop Smoking Permanently

Stop Smoking with Allen Carr (with 70-minute audio CD)

Stop Smoking and Quit E-cigarettes

Your Personal Stop Smoking Plan

How to Stop Your Child Smoking

The Illustrated Easy Way for Women to Stop Smoking

Allen Carr's Quit Drinking Without Willpower

The Illustrated Easy Way to Stop Smoking

Your Personal Stop Drinking Plan

Finally Free!

Allen Carr's Easy Way for Women to Quit Drinking

Smoking Sucks (Parent Guide with 16 page pull-out comic)

The Illustrated Easy Way to Stop Drinking

The Little Book of Quitting

No More Hangovers

How to Be a Happy Non-Smoker

The Easy Way to Mindfulness

No More Ashtrays

Good Sugar Bad Sugar

How to be a Happy Nonsmoker

The Easy Way to Quit Sugar

Allen Carr's Easy Way for Women
to Lose Weight

Lose Weight Now

No More Diets

The Easy Way to Stop Gambling

No More Gambling

No More Worrying

Get Out of Debt Now

No More Debt

The Easy Way to Enjoy Flying

No More Fear of Flying

The Easy Way to Quit Coffee

Burning Ambition

Packing It In The Easy Way
(the autobiography)

Want Easyway on your **smartphone** or **tablet**? Search for "Allen Carr" in your app store.

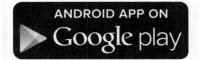
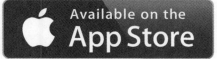

Easyway publications are also available as **audiobooks**. Visit **shop.allencarr.com** to find out more.

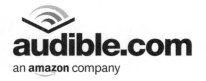

DISCOUNT VOUCHER
for
ALLEN CARR'S
EASYWAY CENTRES

Recover the price of this book when you attend an
Allen Carr's Easyway Centre
anywhere in the world!

Allen Carr's Easyway has a global network of stop
smoking centres where we guarantee you'll find it easy
to stop smoking or your money back.

**The success rate based on this
unique money-back guarantee is over 90%.**

Sessions addressing weight, alcohol and other
drug addictions are also available at certain centres.

When you book your session, mention this
voucher and you'll receive a discount of
the price of this book. Contact your nearest
centre for more information on how the sessions
work and to book your appointment.

**Details of Allen Carr's Easyway
Centres can be found at**
www.allencarr.com

This offer is not valid in conjunction with any other offer/promotion.